Insulin Dependent Diabetes
My First Fifty *Years*

By

John R. Bennett

ISBN: 1-4033-3948-1 (Electronic)
ISBN: 1-4033-3949-X (Softcover)

This book is printed on acid free paper.

1stBooks – rev. 07/23/02

Dedication

This book is dedicated to the memory of Dr. Elliott Proctor Joslin, 1869-1962. His lifetime efforts to conquer 'the gangrene' of insulin dependent diabetes against the odds of alienating himself in his own medical profession are a testament to his inner strength. I met the man on several occasions later in his life, when he visited Camp Joslin in Charlton, Massachusetts, while I was a camper there.

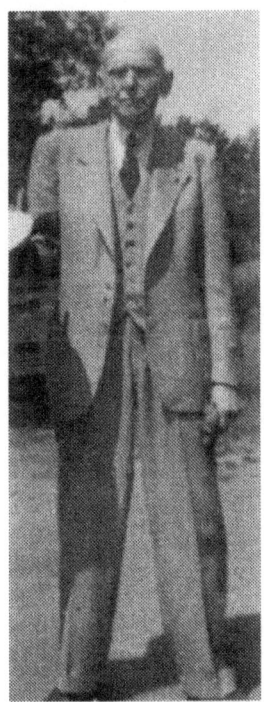

Elliott P Joslin circa 1940

Preface

John Richard Bennett has had insulin dependent (Type-I) diabetes since December 1954. He is a Computer Science Analyst at Brookhaven National Laboratory on Long Island, working there since 1968. Married in 1969, John and his wife Joann have two daughters, Noel (who also has Type-I diabetes) and Krista. Both daughters have children, Heather and Joshua repectively. John's hobbies include camping, kayaking and bicycling.

John is looking forward to the day he receives his "Half Century Award" from the Joslin Clinic in Boston, for combating his diabetes for 50 years. His dream is to be able to ride his bicycle from Riverhead, NY to the Cross Sound Ferry in Orient Point, NY. His wife, driving his vehicle as a sag wagon will take the ferry to New London, Ct. while John kayaks across Long Island Sound. He then intends to continue his bicycling to the Joslin Diabetic Camp in Charlton, Ma. where he will accept his award.

JRB

Table of Contents

Prologue

My hopes for this writing are to give you an insight into my life with diabetes mellitus. Hopefully, you'll see developing trends in diabetes treatment, yet at the same time see that I might have a slight sense of humor. Maybe I won't even bore you to death as you continue reading. My attempt to keep chapters short has actually happened in most cases.

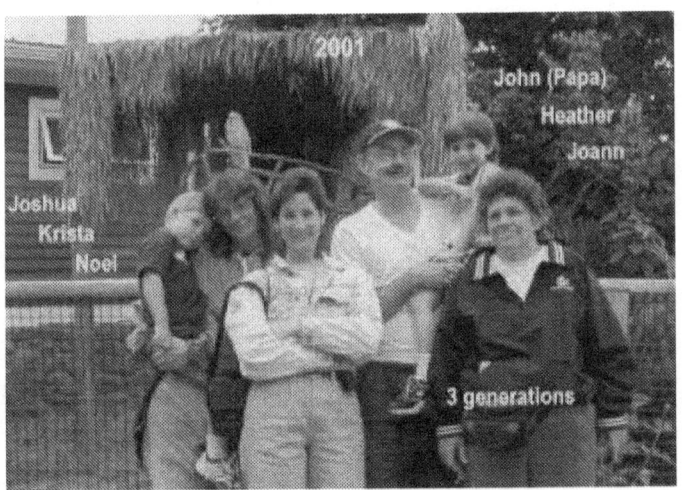

My scrapbook contains fifty years of pictures, articles, newspaper clippings, and a whole lot of notes. Nearly two years have been spent formulating what and how my notes would be transformed to print. As I start this writing, Sept. 2001, I am four weeks short of my fifty-third birthday. In December 2004, I'll look back over fifty years as a Type-I insulin dependent diabetic.

The changes in treatment for this disease are dramatic, but none more so than in the past five years. I remember my first injection using a clear glass syringe with a cobalt blue plunger and a 25 gauge 5/8" stainless steel needle, boiling them every morning before use, even occasionally sharpening the needle for reuse when it dulled. Different types of insulin were in different shaped bottles to tell them apart. Although I was too young to really complain about not being able to eat the candies and desserts, there were many times that envy of the other kids got me down. My mother trained as a dietician to give me a well balanced diet. For years I measured food quantity on a gram scale. It seemed we never ate out. I can't remember where the nearest McDonalds was.

There have been numerous changes in insulin types that I've had to get accustomed to. From U40 in 1954, changing to U80 in 1960, then to U100 in the mid 1970's and finally to Humulin in 1999. For the novice, names were created for the number of units of insulin per milliliter (ml). Example: U40 insulin had 40 units of insulin per ml. Insulin started from a beef source, then a combination of beef and pork, then pork by itself, and of course Humulin is a synthetic (man-made) insulin. The insulin pump I am now wearing uses U100 Humulin Humalog, which is a very fast acting - short life span insulin. That's right; in 2000, after forty-six years I stopped *injecting* insulin.

In the early chapters I have attempted to write from the viewpoint of the youngster I was at the time. It will be clearly marked when I add comments as an adult.

Throughout the book you'll encounter words like hypoglycemia, hyperglycemia, retinopathy, glucose, insulin reaction, etc. For the sake of easy reading, there are no footnotes or emphasis on any of these words. Instead, I have created a glossary with real definitions, not just my slant on them.

I also have a living active faith in God and the Lord Jesus Christ. My life, in my opinion, with its ups and downs, is made both liveable and enjoyable because I was, and still am, daily filled with the Spirit of God.

Hope you enjoy.

John Bennett

Chapter 1
Diagnosis

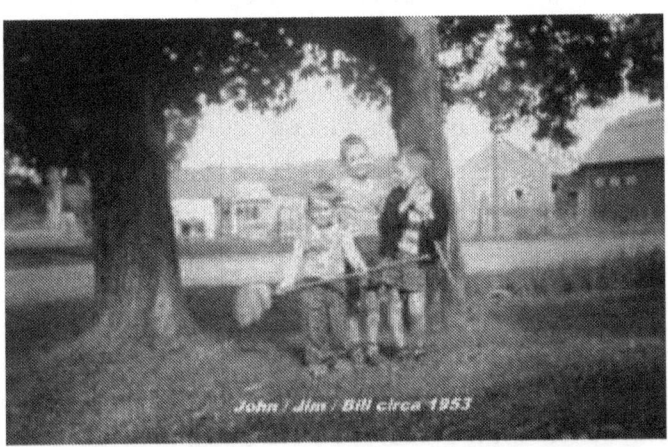

John / Jim / Bill circa 1953

I was born in the St. Albans, Vermont hospital while my parents and two older brothers, Jim & Bill, were living in Georgia Plains, Vt. My Dad was a Baptist Minister; my Mom a school teacher. Although I'm not sure, my younger sister Cheryl, may have been born here too. Dad & Mom moved quite often and before I was six, 1954, we moved to Dickenson Center, which is across Lake Champlain in upper New York State.

In December of that year I got real sick. I don't personally remember my mother taking me to my uncle who was an M.D. and being told that I had diabetes. However, I do remember being so thirsty that I couldn't stop drinking and then making bathroom runs. I was sent to the Joslin Clinic in Boston, specializing in diabetes, where they found my blood sugar reading was over 450 milligram per deciliter (mg/dl). A normal reading is 80-120 mg/dl.

1

Now I'm different. Glass syringe, insert plunger, attach needle, stick it into an orange to practice, draw air into the syringe, agitate insulin so that it's a good mix, wipe the top of the bottle with isopropol alcohol on a cotton ball, inject air into insulin bottle, withdraw insulin, wipe injection site with same cotton ball, inject syringe, dispense insulin, over and over again to the point where you can do it in your sleep. Three times a day I bring out the clinitest kit and take urine tests. If result is high, then I have to check for ketones.

A balance has to be established between Diet, Insulin and Exercise. If tests are high I need to inject more quick acting insulin, U40 Regular, and still include a much longer lasting insulin, U40 NPH. Three times a day for the rest of my life. Maybe I'll get run over by a car, tomorrow. That'll fix 'em. If I go into a low blood sugar condition, called hypoglycemia, no matter where I am or what I'm doing, I have to stop and get some sort of sugar into my body.

Hey, maybe it's not too bad. If I have a test in school, I can fake an insulin reaction and have to go to the nurse's office. No way! That means everyone really will know I'm different.

Across the street from our house was a man who raised turkeys, Don Woods. He would occasionally let my brothers and I ride on the tractor when he took feed into the area where the turkeys were. I had no problem doing this while my brothers were on the tractor with me but I remember a time when I was alone and Don had gotten off the tractor for some reason. Here come *millions* of turkeys trying to *attack me*. It didn't matter that I was on the tractor or that they weren't bothering Don, but I was sure they were after me anyway. Later after my brothers got back from school and laughed at what happened, it was explained to me that my *millions* were actually *hundreds* and the only reason the turkeys crowded around the tractor was because there were too many of them to get to the wagon carrying the grain. Of course I really didn't care that they had all been de-beaked and had their wings clipped. But oh the noise a couple hundred turkeys can make.

My birthday is October 12th so I began 1st grade when I was only five years old. Dad moved us to Starrucca, Pennsylvania where I began fourth grade, so I must have been nine (1957). Most of my growing up years were here. Starrucca is a rural farming community in the north-eastern corner of the state with New York within an hour's drive to the north and to the east.

We made sure that lots of folks knew I had diabetes. I have never been subconscious about what I do to take care of my disease. It's funny. My friends don't care that I have diabetes. Some are oblivious to my 'condition'; others are actually interested and want to know more. The needles really don't hurt; they're tiny. It only takes a few minutes a day. This isn't so bad.

"Mom, it's the ninth inning and I'm up to bat next. No way I can leave now." This is getting worse all the time. But it was supper time and I had to eat on time. If I waited an extra twenty minutes exercising at the same time, I'd be in insulin reaction. They're no fun. The first time I got one, I didn't know what was going on. My body wasn't doing what I thought I was telling it to do. My voice was gone, even though I was trying to scream for help. My knees no longer held me up, but kept buckling. My mouth tasted like it was full of sawdust. It got to the point where I couldn't even remember my name. Mom brought me out of it by forcing me to drink orange juice. About fifteen minutes later I was 'normal' again, but I couldn't remember anything that had happened for the previous half-hour. If someone had seen me would they have thought I was drunk? Embarassing!

"What do you mean I have to learn about the pancreas, and Isles of Langer-whats-its? How do you expect me to do all this? There's no one else around here with diabetes. Even my doctor says so."

3

Yes, I *am* different. A disease called diabetes has me in its hold. But I can and will combat it. I have to take shots to furnish my body with the insulin it no longer produces.

So what. I *can* handle this. There is absolutely no reason to be ashamed I'm diabetic. There is no way I'm going to let diabetes get me down. Excuses and feeling sorry for myself are going to do more harm than good. There will never be a day when I allow my diabetes to be a crutch in my lifestyle. I may have to form habits around it, but I will never allow my disease to stop me from doing anything I want to do.

*   *   *

Now that I'm an adult, I see it was easier for me to learn how to live with diabetes than what it's like as a teenager for example. As a youngster, the peer pressure hasn't really begun. Habits can be formed rather than replaced. My daughter was diagnosed at the age of sixteen and her habits were established and had to be thrown away and new ones created. There have been struggles, however. Doctors who weren't up on diabetes, unexplained patterns of high and low blood sugars, added to my confusion. Things that today, with more and more information available, can be rationalized, weren't even thought about then.

Most children that I've run across have the ability to remember early events in their lives long before I did. Now in 2001, at the age of fifty-three I don't believe myself old but, if the shoe fits…A friend of mine recently promised me, 'It's not Alzheimer's, it's old-timers'.

The name Joslin is going to be mentioned quite frequently. My training began at the Joslin Clinic but continued at the Joslin Diabetic Camp in Charlton, Massachusetts. I will always have fond memories of Dr. Elliott Proctor Joslin, whom I personally met and talked to, and for whom the camp was named, where I spent so many summers of

4

my life and still go to for visits. One of my best friends, Paul Madden, who has taken a career as a Diabetes advocate, lecturing and advising, still spends most of his summers taking a leadership role at the camp.

Isaiah 30:20,21-KJV Although the Lord gives you the bread of adversity and the water of affliction, your teachers will be hidden no more; with your own eyes you will see them. Whether you turn to the right or to the left, your ears will hear a voice behind you, saying, "This is the way; walk in it."

Chapter 2
Training

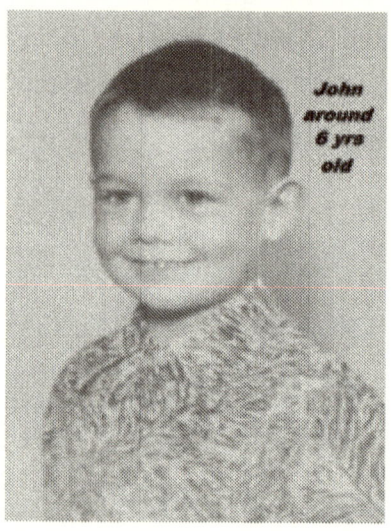

Monday - Six years old, in the middle of winter; I could be home sleigh riding. Instead I'm in Boston at the Joslin Clinic learning about diabetes. This place is huge.

Yesterday, we (my class and I) learned about what insulin was, how it worked, the differences in types of insulin, and why I was on a combination of 'regular' and 'NPH'. We learned the necessity of boiling our syringe and needle before each use, how to draw a mixture of insulin, and practiced injecting an orange because its skin has the same resistance as our own.

Tuesday - Today we're learning about using Clinitest kits: the correct number of drops of urine combined with the correct number of drops of water, dropping in the Clinitest tablet, watching the fizz then waiting for the color to tell us the result. Because urine is part of body waste, this result was telling us what amount of sugar was spilling into the urine within the last four hours. Negative (a blue color) meant we weren't spilling any sugar, while 4+ (orange) showed that we could have from a moderate blood sugar to a high blood sugar. There were also ranges in the middle. If we were negative, our insulin dose was considered sufficient (a grown up word for OK). If 4+ we also had to test for ketones. Joslin told us what these were but I didn't care. I knew the word, knew how to test for them, knew to call my doctor if the test appeared positive. That's going to have to be enough.

We were warned about complications from long term uncontrolled diabetes, but I guess I wasn't listening to that either. No way was I going to get anything else. Why won't they let me go play baseball, instead? Mom's here somewhere taking a course on what I'm supposed to eat and when.

Oh yeah, I was given my own gram scale this morning. Did you know a medium sized potato weighs around 60 grams. Doctor Root has given me a 1200 calorie diet and it actually looks pretty good. Mom says I won't have any trouble with it because she hasn't found any food yet that I won't eat, even vegetables. I eat six times a day now, isn't that great? Breakfast, lunch, and dinner, plus a snack mid morning, another mid afternoon and a third before I go to bed. This is to keep my carbohydrate intake as regular as possible throughout the entire day. I only take one shot in the morning, right now: four units of 'regular' and sixteen units of 'NPH' before breakfast. The regular works real fast but doesn't last long. The NPH doesn't start working for a while but lasts a lot longer. Once I get out of the hospital, I'm told that the amount of insulin may go down when I start to get more exercise. To keep everything in balance my exercise is supposed to be scheduled for the same times each day and stop after a certain amount of time.

Wednesday - You should have seen what I just did. I went to the lab this morning to have a blood test. The nurse took it from my arm and while we were waiting to get the result, she taught me how to draw my own blood. There was a small tube about a foot long, a pipette (that's a long slender glass tube), a lancet and a mirror. I swabbed one of my earlobes with isopropol alcohol, pricked it with the lancet, and put one end of the tube onto the pipette with the other end in my mouth. Sucking on the tube and pinching my earlobe with my fingers, the blood went right up into the pipette. When it was full, we emptied it into a glass tube with a stopper, then put it into a centrifuge. A centrifuge is a machine that spins in a circle with clips on it to hold the tubes. This keeps the blood from coagulating (another grown up word that means it stops it from getting thick - like cream on top of a bottle of milk). How they test the blood is a mystery. I wasn't allowed to watch that, but a man came back and said my test was 120. We were taught that a good result was 110-130.

This afternoon was a little scary. A nurse was showing Mom and I what I would look like, act like and feel like when I went into an insulin reaction. That's when my blood sugar level goes too low. When it gets real low my body starts to secrete adrenalin because it doesn't know how to handle it. The nurse gave me an injection of regular insulin and started taking blood sugars every five minutes. After about ten minutes I started feeling funny. My sugar was 85, I was starting to sweat, and my tongue felt too large. When it got down to 60 my words started to slur and my legs wouldn't hold me up any more. By the time it dropped to 50 I don't remember much except Mom made me drink a glass of orange juice. I felt better about five minutes later. My blood sugar went back up to 120 and everything was back to normal.

Thursday - Can you imagine that a colored pair of socks can cause all sorts of problems for a diabetic? Neither could I. But now my socks are supposed to be white cotton so that no dye can get into my feet. Poor circulation can be a big problem. It can lead to all sorts of things. Mom and I are supposed to find me a doctor who knows about diabetes. We live in a farming community in northern New York State and Mom thinks that might be a problem.

Mom's been great. She and I have been praying together a lot this week. But she doesn't seem to be as excited to go home as I am. She tells me over and over that I need to have enough courage to handle the responsibility. Don't worry, Mom, I'll handle it.

Friday - We go home this afternoon. Wow! Prior to leaving we're learning how to increase my diet when it's necessary. I've learned more about calories and grams and vegetables than I'll ever need to know. A 3% vegetable, like lettuce, can be eaten almost as a free food. Vegetables like spinach are 6%. It's funny about carrots. Raw, they're 3%; cooked they're 6%. Potatoes are 20%. The percentage stands for the amount of carbohydrate content by weight. All foods are broken down by the body into different things like protein, fat and carbohydrate. We had to learn what each did, and what foods created what, so that we could calculate how much insulin to take every day.

Mom and I met Dr. Priscilla White today. What a nice lady. We talked about enrolling me at the Joslin Camp in Charlton, Massachusetts next summer. It's a camp for diabetic boys that teaches them (she means me) how to interact with other kids and stay on my regime (that means my balance of diet, insulin, and exercise).

Finally; we're on our way home!

I should have listened more in class. I'm having way too many insulin reactions. Maybe this is what Mom was worried about. I'll try harder.

*   *   *

The Joslin Clinic, in my humble opinion (IMHO), is probably the greatest training facility for youngsters or adults for diabetic training.

The staff has always been superb in their knowledge and bedside manner; the doctors, well known in their fields, are both personable and willing to give of their time. Many thanks, Joslin.

Through the intervening years insulin reactions were too numerous to even count. My main problem was that I was an exercise junky. Once we had moved to Pennsylvania, sports, even though I wasn't very good at them, consumed me. I constantly argued with my Mother about leaving a ball game "just to go home and eat". Or why couldn't I ride my bike up to the dairy farm before supper to help milk the cows? Just because I wouldn't get back before seven o'clock shouldn't make any difference.

As a parent-now a grandparent- I see, too late, the aggravation we can cause in our parents lives. I've never seen a more concerned, loving, caring individual than my Mother. God bless you, Mom.

Ephesians 6:4-NIV Fathers, do not exasperate your children; instead, bring them up in the training and instruction of the Lord.

Chapter 3
Camp Life

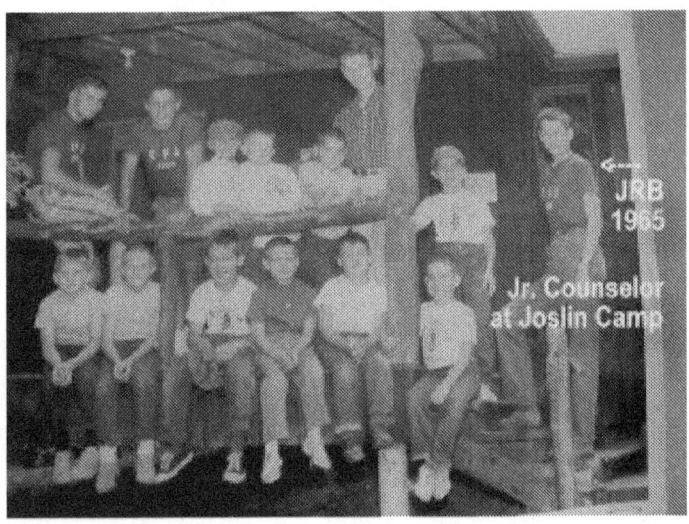

1955 - Wow! What a great place. Getting my trunk into my cabin by 9AM and being introduced to all the other guys in the cabin we easily make friends and started doing things together. Cabin seven is for six and seven year olds and is my first cabin. Cabins seven and eight make up Junior Division and we have our own special area for games. There is special diabetes instruction every day. Our day starts at 7AM with specs at the lab (urine tests 4 times a day as well as blood tests 3 days a week). We even have to collect 24 hour specimens twice a week. After specs we line up at the infirmary to get our morning shots. By this time I have started injecting two shots a day, one in the morning and one before bed.

We have every kind of sport imaginable. My favorite is hiking to Dresser Hill. You have to realize what Dresser Hill is for this to make any sense. It's a place where they make homemade ice cream, about four-and-one-half miles from camp. We would ride in the van, get our ice cream, be driven half way back, then walk the rest of the way. Most of the time we would sing camp songs at the top of our lungs. Of course, we do that in the mess hall after each meal too. Even sing grace before each meal.

There is Indian Counsel. I am a Mohawk. The last week of camp we have the Sioux - Mohawk wars (don't tell anyone, but it's a form of capture the flag). Once a week we troupe at night to the counsel fire and listen to the chiefs tell us what we need to do during the week. My war club passed the rock test the first time around.

1956 - Now I'm in Cabin Eight. Two campers from last year are here with me again. I was only homesick two nights this time. Last year I was just a kid. I spend almost every less-active period this year learning how to paddle a canoe and will receive my Canoeing Merit Badge by the end of session. We're making lanyards in arts and crafts.

1957 - I'm back at Joslin in Cabin Six and am learning how to shoot a bow and arrow but I still love paddling a canoe and rowing. I'm learning how to play basketball the right way. I still love playing baseball, but I guess I'm not very good at it. There's a new room with a ping-pong table and we're having a lot of fun. On Sunday mornings we go out and have services at the Chapel in the Woods. My diet has been increased again. I'm now getting 1500 calories per day. I'm taking 12 units of regular and 18 units of NPH in the morning and 2 units of NPH at night.

My parents struggle to allow me to go to camp each summer. Arriving and signing in, I heard the Camp Director explaining to my father the breakdown of camp costs. One item was a laundry bill. It was a minimal amount but as a young boy I thought I could save my Dad that expense. So I stayed in the same clothes for most of the session only cleaning them during shower time. Once Dad picked me up at the end of session, he was quite perturbed at me. He had already prepaid the laundry fee when he dropped me off.

1958 - Mom and Dad are sending me to Pennsylvania's Camp Firefly this summer.

1959 - This year I am going to Camp NYDA in New York.

1960 - Cabin three. I think this is the greatest cabin. You're already at the top of the hill and it's easier to get everywhere. The mess hall is only forty feet away. I've learned several different swimming strokes this year and I'm now in pool 2. That means no matter where you jump in from the dock it's over your head. Both my insulin and diet have increased. I'm now taking an extra pre-supper insulin injection. One of the campers threatened to run away last night. His counselor found him under the cabin after supper. I can't imagine anyone wanting to leave camp to go home. I'd stay all summer if they'd let me. I met Mr. & Mrs. Perkins again this year. Mr. Perkins maintains the camp grounds and Mrs. Perkins works in the kitchen. One of the counselors brought his dog "Perky" to camp with him. Of course, the song 'A Little Black Dog' had the dog's name changed from Bingo to Perky.

1961 - Dad couldn't send me to camp this summer.

1962 - Cabin 1. What a great bunch of guys here this year. We're scheduled to go mountain climbing on Mount Monadnock in New Hampshire next week. Shot my first rifle this morning. For some reason the camp isn't going to offer riflery any more; something about too many advocates objecting. Met a couple of counselors from Africa this year who play soccer and know Pele of the New York Cosmos and a retired top seeded tennis player by the name of Billy Talbert. He gave a clinic at the tennis courts. After seeing me serving some balls, he approached me, put his arm around my shoulders and said, "Son, I think you better find a different sport. This one isn't yours". What do you think he meant by that?

1963 - I'm in the Senior Division, Tent-A. It's been a great summer but I'm sad because it's the last year I can be a camper. Thinking back over the years I've been coming here, I see that most of the sports I know how to play I learned here. Other activities, like working with my hands, learning chess, canoeing, kayaking, archery, hiking all had their beginnings here. I'm going to be sorry to leave.

1964 - My application to become a Counselor in Training (CIT) was approved by the Unitarian Universalist Womens Federation. I'm back at Joslin helping kids get through the same doubts and fears that I once had. Because I had to adjust to life as a diabetic, I can share actual experiences. Not only do I know the apprehensions they are experiencing, but I can share what does or doesn't work to alleviate those apprehensions. My cabin is Cabin 7 which has the youngest campers and is part of Junior Division. Did I really look this young when I started coming to camp here?

1965 - This is my first year as a Junior Counselor in Cabin 8. It's the third week of camp but I'm no longer at camp. Instead, I've been admitted to Worcester General Hospital. This morning at 4AM I went to the infirmary at camp with the worst stomach cramps I have ever had. The pain started in the center of my abdomen but slowly moved to the right side. It was late in the afternoon when I was put into the

14

ambulance, driven to the hospital and diagnosed with appendicitis. Of course, my summer is being cut short.

*   *   *

During one of the summers I was at camp we were allowed to bring our bicycles. I had learned to ride while we lived in Dickenson Center, N.Y. It was actually my brother's bike but I used it more than he did. There were two old tractor tires on the front lawn filled with dirt where Mom planted flowers. Our porch was raised with four steps and had lattice work from the bottom of the porch to the ground except for one area right next to the steps. I would climb onto the nearest tire to be able to get on the bike and ride around the yard. Stopping was a different matter. I would ride right up to the steps and just let the bike go under the porch. This is the one area there was no longer any lattice.

I met Doctor Joslin while at camp one summer. What a fantastic person. Even though he walked slowly and with a cane he talked to each one of us, giving advice and a word of encouragement. One summer when I was in Senior Division I learned he had passed away during the previous winter. There was to be a memorial service at the Oxford Cemetery where he was buried and I was going to be able to attend. What a privilege.

*   *   *

There are literally dozens of diabetic camps populating the United States. Some are co-ed while others are for either boys or girls. Growing up I needed to know that I wasn't alone in what was going on in my life. I spent seven years as a camper at the Joslin Diabetic Camp for boys in Charlton, Massachusetts. My parents sent me to Camp Firefly in Pennsylvania one summer and Camp NYDA in New

York, another. They were both closer to home but after my first year at Joslin, nothing else seemed to compare.

There is nothing to compare to camp life where everyone in your cabin, including most of the counselors, have diabetes. Once I became an age where I could no longer be a camper I became a counselor in training and then a junior counselor. My second year ended rather suddenly when I was rushed to the hospital with appendicitis. That winter I met my future wife and now only occasionally go back to Joslin.

In my scrapbook are many letters from doctors at the Joslin Clinic; Dr. Howard Root, Dr. Priscilla White, Dr. Leo Krall, and I even have one addressed to my parents signed by Dr. Elliott P. Joslin dated September 24, 1957. My parents were being encouraged by Dr. Joslin to allow me to be an active inquisitive 'lad' and with the help of diabetic camp life he foresaw me growing up into a 'well-rounded' *healthy* young man.

There were many friends I met at Camp Joslin, but only two I've really kept up with. One is Paul Madden, who was never in my cabin (don't expect me to admit I'm older than he is). Paul has become Special Assistant to the President, Joslin Diabetes Center. A great speaker and fellow diabetic, he's a really great guy. He still spends an enormous amount of time at the camp. Joslin Clinic awards the 'Half Century Award' to those Type-I diabetics that have lived with the disease for fifty years. It is my wish that Paul be present at camp to personally give me my Half Century Award.

The second person I want to mention is not diabetic nor did he ever attend the camp as either a camper or counselor. His name is Peter Starkus. Peter took over for Mr. Perkins in charge of grounds maintenance. A plumber by trade, who is also the town's Plumbing Inspector, Peter single-handedly put together the new water pumping station at camp. Peter allows me to come up once in a while and give a helping hand trimming trees, helping erect cabins, or whatever he is working on.

I can't begin to tell you how many great people comprise an institution like Camp Joslin, but my hat is off to you two gentlemen.

Genesis 32:21-NIV So Jacob's gifts went on ahead of him, but he himself spent the night in the camp.

Chapter 4
Accident Prone?

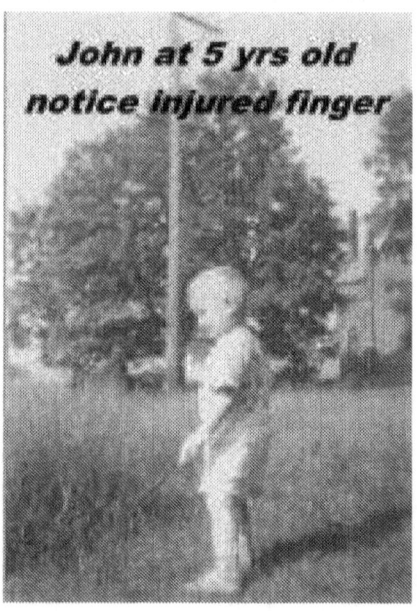

John at 5 yrs old notice injured finger

Once I had reached the age of seven, I felt my Father had some problems with our relationship. Maybe because my diabetes tended my Mother to 'show favoritism' in his eyes—I can't be certain. My Dad is no longer here to ask. Prior to my moving out of the house, first to go live on a dairy farm at age eleven, then when I got my job and then got married, he and I were at odds with each other. Dad always complained that I was getting into stuff and finally decided I was accident prone.

When I was five years old I followed my father into the basement of our house in Georgia Plains, Vermont. Always inquisitive, I wanted to know what the funny looking thing with wheels and belt were. At that instant the electric water pump turned on and my finger was pinched between the roller and belt. Ending up in the hospital, they had to sew the tip of my left middle finger back onto my finger. Later I would have no feeling in the tip of that finger and yet there were two healthy growing fingernails one on top of each other.

I have two older brothers, Jim and Bill, and a younger sister Cheryl. One day I was hit in the head by a tree limb. Jim recollects this differently than I do and I'll use his version.

"I remember a clear day, perhaps windy, and the tree limb just fell. We were all three playing in the yard, and you were the one to get hit. I always assigned that to you being the one accident prone."

Dad's always been glad I've got a hard head.

Dad was a Baptist Minister but his pay wasn't very much in those days and he would take on extra side jobs. We had recently moved from Vermont to Dickenson Center, NY and he was painting a store. They were tearing apart an old barn nearby and, again being inquisitive, I found an upstairs haymow with a swing door in one of the walls. Of course, Dad was hollering at me to get out of the barn. But instead of walking down what was left of the stairs, I jumped out the hay door. When I walked up to Dad, there was a piece of lumber attached to the bottom of my right foot with a nail sticking through the foot. I think the shots they later gave me were worse than the nail.

Sharing a bedroom, another time my brothers and I were jumping back and forth between beds. We had recently hacksawed off the round brass head and footboard framing but, as yet, hadn't capped the ends. You guessed it. Another hospital visit and stitches one-half inch from my right eye. Boy did we all get hollered at for that one.

When I was eight, just before I started fourth grade, we moved to Starrucca, Pennsylvania—real dairy farms and coal furnaces. I found a friend in our coal-delivery man and on occasion was allowed to ride in his 10 ton Mack truck to pick up coal from the coal mines in

Carbondale. In the winter after coming back to deliver the coal, we had to pick through the first two inches of ice to get to the coal.

Every year on the last day of school, the students were allowed to ride their bikes to school. Our school was in Thompson, four-and-a-half miles away. I was in sixth grade when I decided I wanted to ride to school. My teacher, knowing about my diabetes, wasn't too sure about the idea but my parents allowed it and I haven't stopped riding distances since. In later years I found inter-town rides mundane—inter-state rides were much more challenging.

One of the church deacons had a small grove of Christmas trees he raised on the hill behind the parsonage. One winter the kids in town decided to go sleigh riding on that hill. The problem was it had rained during the night and there was a thin layer of ice on the snow. It took nearly thirty minutes getting half way up the hill before we all realized it wasn't worth it and started coming back down. No way was I going to walk. Getting on my sled I started down the hill. I found out real quick, I couldn't steer. Trying to negotiate a turn, my legs came off the sled and promptly slammed into one of the Christmas trees. Guess who won that battle. My cast started chest high and went down both legs, even covering most of my feet. I can't remember Dad ever being so mad. Maybe because he was actually charged for the Christmas tree.

You'll have to make your own decision as to whether you think I'm accident prone or not. But throughout all of my hospital stays or immobility, I never had a problem with my diabetes. Taking more insulin when I was inactive or even when I was sick became second nature. As my experience with diabetes increased so did my willpower to be in control of it. Doctors have remarked on numerous occasions as to how fast and well I had healed without any infections. After a while, I no longer became elated with this kind of comment but more or less expected it of myself. I remembered my comment to

Mom before leaving the training session at the Joslin Clinic, "I'll handle it".

*   *   *

Just prior to getting married my Dad and I got close again. The reasons we gave each other for our antagonism are too personal to go into. But for the next several years our relationship grew. I was the first sibling to get married and Joann and I were married in her church by my father. We have pictures of Dad holding his first grandchild, Noel. Just after our second child, Krista, was born, Dad went to live with Jesus Christ.

No matter what you've decided about my being accident prone, I've filled my life with all sorts of exciting things. I've ridden horses, driven tractors, been snow mobiling over 80 miles per hour, taken interstate bicycle rides, kayaked on class 4 rivers, descended Mt. Monadnock in New Hampshire with full backpack, even ascended the Washington Monument on crutches. Besides normal childhood diseases I've been diagnosed with diabetes (age 6), had appendicitis (age 17), went through seven laser treaments for retinopathy (age 28), double bypass open heart surgery (age 51) and kidney stones (age 52 & 53).

I just can't wait to see what happens next.

Proverbs 24:10-KJV If thou faint in the day of adversity, thy strength is small.

Chapter 5
Driver's License

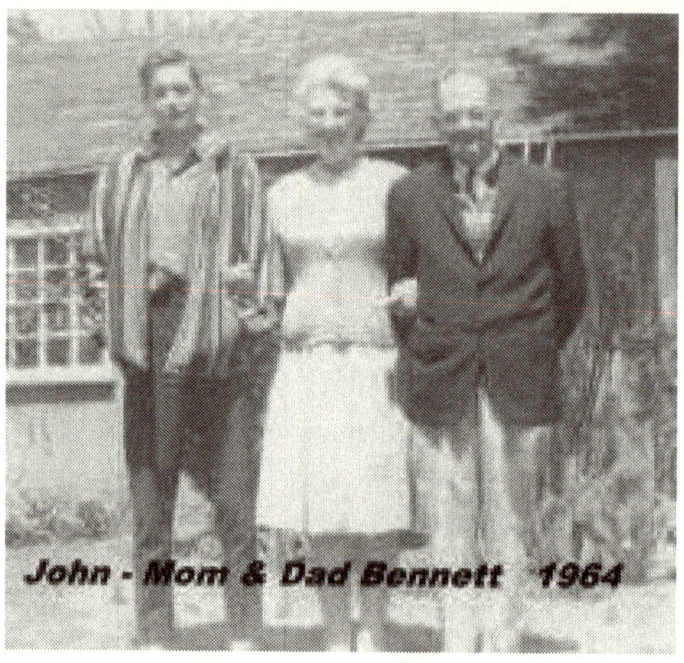

John - Mom & Dad Bennett   1964

Insurance for individuals with no physical ailment seems to be taken for granted. My experience has taught me this is not so for individuals with diabetes.

My parents moved from Pennsylvania to East Marion, Long Island the summer of 1965 while I was a counselor at Camp Joslin. When they wrote and told me, I was first astonished because I hadn't heard them mention even the possiblity of this. Secondly, I was mad. Living in Pennsylvania, a youngster is allowed his driving permit at the age of sixteen and I had already applied for my permit. Now I had to start all over again.

Coming home from camp, I was healing from my appendicitis operation. Not being able to move around much for a couple of weeks left me time to call the Motor Vehicle Dept. to have them send me paperwork for obtaining my learner's permit. For once I was almost ready to lie about my diabetes. Prior to being issued a permit, I had to prove that I was on an insurance policy. Applying for insurance caused me all sorts of hassles. The instructions stated that I was required to get letters from two physicians attesting to the fact that my diabetes would not affect my safe handling of a motor vehicle.

The family's personal physician had no problem with this as long as the permit stated that I had diabetes and was insulin dependent. Dad called another doctor in town, then went to pick up his letter. My father and I didn't see eye to eye on a lot of things, but our response to that letter was a united front. The doctor had stated that because I had the possiblity of becoming unconscious behind the wheel it was *his expert opinion* that I should not be issued a driver's license. We found out later he had written similar letters before and did not advocate any diabetic holding a driver's license.

I finally got the letter I required from the Joslin Clinic. It angers me that there was such discrimination. I argue that controlled diabetics have less likelihood of being unconscious than an epileptic or a drunk. People who occasionally go into epileptic 'fits' have the same problem as the diabetic with insurance but an otherwise normal individual who drinks is never screened. Where on a driver's license application does it read, "Do you ever use alcoholic beverages?"

Living on a dairy farm, I had driven farm vehicles for years. Most farm lads begin driving tractors before they are ten years old. I'd driven caterpillars as well as tractor trailers before I was sixteen (off the road, of course). I took pride in how I was in control of my diabetes. Testing several times a day, taking my shots at the prescribed times, eating my meals when I should, very seldom seeing the insulin reactions any more and then only after heavy physical exercise, IMHO driving didn't pose a problem to anyone. How can I convince anyone?

*   *   *

I left home to live on the dairy farm when I was eleven. It was on the farm I learned to get up early, 4:30 AM, to help milk cows. It was my job to put the milkers together and bring them from the milk house into the barn. There was a bull in the barn that I was warned to stay away from. He gave me my first introduction to the reproduction process.

He also scared me half to death one morning. Carrying the milkers into the barn, I had stopped to turn on the lights and I could see the bull in the middle of the aisle with his stanchion around his neck and the chains that would have anchored the stanchion to the floor and higher beams just dangling. As soon as he saw me he charged. Leaving the milkers right where they were I dove into the saw-dust bin and just kept climbing. We were finally able to corner him at the back of the barn by driving the tractor down the center aisle. Once someone was able to grab his nose ring he was docile as could be.

Norm Glover, the farm owner's son, taught me how to make root beer one summer. We used old quart beer bottles we picked up at a supermarket and sterilized, added yeast to the root beer mix and we'd make, bottle, and cork about twenty-four quarts at a time. Then we'd box the bottles and store them in an empty upstairs room on the farm until they had aged.

One hot summer afternoon after loading two wagons with baled hay, Norm and I came to the kitchen to get something to drink. My blood sugar was low and a glass of root beer sounded just right.

24

Going into the refrigerator I found a bottle that had previously been opened and was nearly empty.

My father, a Baptist minister, walked in the door as I started drinking straight from the beer bottle. I immediately had to convince him that I wasn't drinking beer, or he wouldn't have let me stay on the farm. As we're "visiting" we started hearing what we thought was a car backfiring. First one, then seconds later another. Within three minutes we had lost count. Twenty minutes later we watched as root beer began dripping from the kitchen ceiling. Maybe we used a little too much yeast? What a mess.

Norm and I joined a men's bowling league in Hancock, N.Y., which was about fourteen miles from the farm by road. On Wednesday nights during the winter months we'd let Norm's mother & father finish milking without us. When there was snow on the ground it was easier and faster to drive the snowmobile over the mountain to the bowling alley instead of going by car on the roads. The only problem was when it started getting cold and we had to come back over that mountain with the wind blowing over thirty miles an hour and a wind-chill factor of -20. We had many bone chilling nights coming over that mountain.

*   *   *

Getting insurance for a driver's license is one of many bureaucratic problems facing a diabetic that as an adult I can empathize with. Health insurance can cause the same problems. I've been turned down for health insurance policies because of "previous existing conditions". Insurance companies have come a long way since I had these hassles, but not far enough.

Yet, maybe, you need to hear the other side of the argument. Statistics prove that the standard ratios of accidents to number of drivers increases when the number of drivers with diabetes who have accidents is factored in. You can argue that statistics can be manipulated, and I won't dispute it. However, as a controlled diabetic I am appalled at the number of individuals with diabetes who first, are not controlled, and second, don't put any effort into attempting to be. This is what jacks up the statistics against diabetic drivers, not the insurance companies themselves.

I have *NEVER* used diabetes as an excuse for anything. I have *NEVER* been ashamed to tell anyone that I had diabetes. My prayer is that I *NEVER* will. During the latter part of 1998, I became aware that as a diabetic I could receive a 'handicapped' parking sticker for my automobile. I didn't have to have an amputated leg or be half blind, but, just have diabetes. Growing up with diabetes has made me a healthier person for it. I eat a balanced diet, get physical exercise of some sort or another every day. There's no way I intend to take advantage of 'the system' just to save myself a few steps getting into a building. Persons having complications from diabetes that require these stickers have my wholehearted support. But they could have gotten them because of their condition alone, not because it was diabetes induced.

Judges 11:17-NIV Give us permission to go through your country...

Chapter 6
New Job

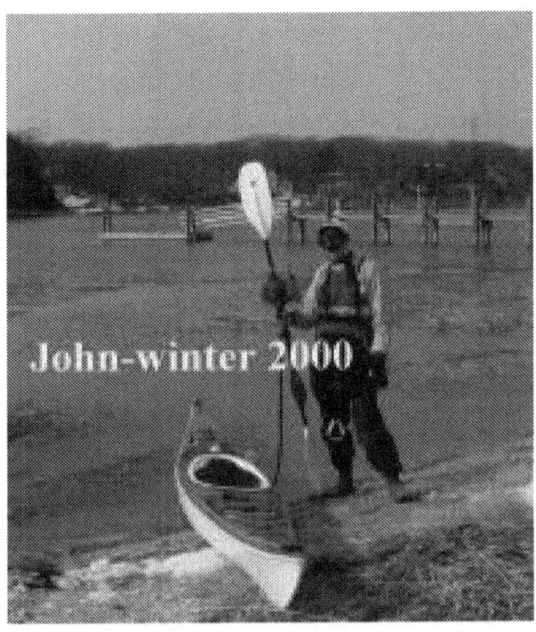

John-winter 2000

During the winter of 1967 our church youth group had finished decorating the Fellowship Hall for our annual Christmas party. We were in the middle of a severe snowstorm and the roads were barely passable. Being one of the youth leaders, I had just completed driving three of the youngsters and another leader to their homes and I was now alone in the vehicle. While returning home I was unable to negotiate a curve in the road and had an automobile accident. There were four other separate accident victims in the Emergency Room when I arrived. My doctor had already arrived but there were no available nurses to assist with the stitches necessary in my knee. So I ended up assisting. I was sent home the next morning but had to return a week later. My knee had swollen and was severely infected. This was the first time I remember fearing that perhaps I was remiss in maintaining total control of my diabetes. A couple of days later, still in the hospital, I was again on the road to recovery.

One afternoon about 2:30 PM I noticed one of the Aides coming into work. She had a beautiful smile and I wanted to meet her. Once I had, it was obvious I was hooked. Maybe she wasn't a beauty queen but I found she was more beautiful on the inside than anyone I had ever met. She and I really hit it off. Joann introduced me to her parents, and the next summer, I started working for her father in his lawn care and maintenance business. Her Dad treated me royally from the first day. Whenever I needed extra carbohydrate we would go to our favorite snack shop and have coffee and a snack or lunch. After two weeks he could tell when I started going low and would 'take a break'. My involvement with Joann increased and we began talking about futures.

Before we could get married I needed a full time job with medical benefits. I applied at Brookhaven National Laboratory (BNL) in Upton, New York, and was interviewed for a 'Computer Operator' position. As an equal opportunity employer Brookhaven had no problem with my application stating I had diabetes. I passed my aptitude test, was hired, and began working straight days until I was trained and then was moved to a team working Dupont shifts. This is seven days working 4PM to midnight, two days off, seven days working midnight to 8AM with three days off, then seven days working 8AM to 4PM with two days off. I couldn't get my diabetes regulated working Dupont. After six weeks I had lost fifteen pounds and was having problems with high blood sugars. My doctor wrote me a medical excuse to get me back on a straight shift. I came to enjoy the 4PM to midnight shift with its 15% differential. I was on this shift for nearly five years.

Having previously graduated from the Electronic Programming Institute of Smithtown I had some computer programming training. This became extremely valuable when I interviewed for a position as a member of the Systems Programming Group within our building. I was only the second operator to advance from Operations to another group within the computing facility.

You old-timer computer literates might develop nostalgia reading this. My computer job started with "tab" machines: key punch, printers, reproducers, collators, sorters, all using (or creating) old-fashioned punched IBM data cards. The holes in these cards comprised 'hollerith' code. I became proficient at reading this code just by looking at the punched holes in the cards. If you remember a couple of years ago, Florida had a problem in an election tabulating returns because of a "chad" problem. Chad is the name given the tiny pieces that are removed from the data cards. We worked with Calcomp equipment and I became an expert with India Ink graphs. Storage was comprised of either magnetic tape or hard disk. The first tapes I worked with were 200 bits per inch (bpi). Other density included 556 bpi and 1600 bpi. Later tape drives were 6250 bpi. Disks were large and cumbersome. We backed up data at that time to large removable disks, the Control Data 841 diskpack. Note: today, the PC in my home has more data storage than twenty of these diskpacks put together and I can hold my PC disk in the palm of my hand.

I have many fond memories from my experience of working at Brookhaven National Laboratory since April 1968. While a computer operator for the first six years, during the time I was working the midnight to eight shift, the shift was slowly coming to an end. The computer center had a raised floor with air conditioning coming through vents in the tiles. Around six-thirty I noticed what looked like animal hair coming from one of the vents. But it seemed as if it were stationary rather than floating up into the room. Grabbing a floor puller I removed a 24" x 24" section of flooring and a cat jumped out and scampered away. A few minutes later, one of the programming staff approached us asking where we had found his cat. He had been working late the night before, fell asleep in his office and the cat that he had brought from home, just to have company, had escaped from his office.

One of the perks working for Brookhaven during the period we had computers from Digital Equipment Corp. was semi-annual Digital Equipment Corp. Users Society (DECUS) meetings at various locations across the country. Paul Kessler, Ed Brosnan, and I decided to go to one of these conventions in Atlanta. Seeking to save some money for the laboratory and to get a new experience, we decided to go by Amtrac rather than flying. Reserving sleeper car rooms, we were ready for the trip. These rooms contained a fold out bed that, once down, covered the room's toilet and seat. Everyone but me believed there to be no way to get the bed down from inside with the door closed. Of course, being skinny and taking up the challenge I entered the room and closed the door. Several minutes later I opened the door from the inside while lying on the bed. I've never told anyone how I was able to do it.

At least twice during my life at Brookhaven I have been tempted to change positions. Sending out resumes on one occasion in the North Carolina area where Joann and I originally felt we would like to retire, I communicated with a company who wanted to interview me for a position. Only a few close friends at work knew about this. Receiving a phone call from a Mr. Delrae, I was engrossed in my conversation when he asked my pardon for a few moments. Seconds later Paul Kessler entered my office and, seeing I was on the phone, excused himself but before leaving said "I see you're on the phone with Mr. Delrae, I don't want to interrupt". It took nearly five seconds before it dawned on me he was pulling a prank. Later Paul, Ed Brosnan and I had a real laugh at my gullibility.

Payback is beautiful. During a DECUS trip Paul took on his own, another coworker and I rigged Paul's office. We removed all the flourescent light bulbs from his fixtures and left them stored in a box in his office. We wrapped an old fishing lure in an Italian newspaper and left it on his desk. Upon his return, of course his light switch didn't work. In the dim light, as he started unwrapping the fishing lure we began playing our cassette version of the theme to "The Godfather".

In over thirty years of working at Brookhaven I can only remember once where my diabetes really caused a ruckus. My stomach was upset that day coming to work. We had a group meeting scheduled at 10AM. I lost my breakfast at 9:55AM, yet instead of getting some carbohydrates into my system I went to the meeting. Half way through the meeting I realized I was beginning hypoglycemia and made another *BIG* mistake. The meeting should be over soon and I'd wait 'til it was over. I was unconscious five minutes later. Coworkers called the BNL EMTs, but they were not prepared for a diabetic emergency. They prepared to transport me to the hospital which is a fifteen minute ride. I've never been leery about telling coworkers about my diabetes and one of them really came through for me. The EMTs were not allowed to give an unconscious person anything by mouth. Now that there are better alternatives, I whole-heartedly agree, but I had previously told Karl Abrams that in an emergency, he could force me to drink orange juice. Five minutes later I was fine, except for the self-incrimination and the embarassment knowing I had perpetuated a bad situation.

This incident took place in the mid 1970's. I don't believe at that time, items such as glucotabs even existed. These are tablets of fast acting carbohydrate that can be taken without drawing anyones attention and would have been ideal in this situation. There also was no 'Glucagon Emergency Kit'. This is a small plastic container holding a syringe and glucagon solution that can be injected into any subcutaneous area of the body. Fluids *should not* be administered to an unconscious patient. This injection would have had the same effect as the orange juice without any possiblity of choking the patient. Since this incident there has been more formal training of EMT staff and they are now prepared for this type of emergency. To date, there are thirty+ insulin dependent diabetics who work at Brookhaven. I now carry a tube of glucotabs in my pocket at all times and have a Glucagon Emergency Kit in my desk with instructions how to use it. There are also numerous coworkers who are now trained on how to administer the injection.

Here's an incident on the more humorous side; at least as far as I'm concerned. There were many years when going to work early in the morning was a must to be able to test new code on a computer before it was required to be back online for 'prime-time' (08:30-17:00). Being at work at five or six in the morning was not uncommon. On this particular occasion there was a young lady coworker sharing computer time. Once I booted the computer to bring it back online, I would take my insulin injection and go to the cafeteria for breakfast. Doing this hundreds of times in the past it never dawned on me that someone might be terrified of needles. Sitting at my desk with my office door open, this young lady walked into my office just as I was injecting myself. Turning as I heard her gasp, she was clutching her stomach with one hand and her mouth with the other. The look in her eyes convinced me she was about to faint. Do you think maybe I should have shut the door first?

In April, 2001 I celebrated my thirty-second year at Brookhaven. There's a magic number here at Brookhaven. When employees reach the magic number with either thirty-five consecutive years of service or have reached the age of fifty-five, they are able to retire and receive their medical insurance for life at the rate they were contributing at the time of their retirement. This magic number is seventy and is the addition of number of consecutive years service added to their age. April, 2003 will be my thirty-fifth anniversary. October, 2003 will be my fifty-fifth birthday. I intend to retire in 2003 while my wife and I are young enough to take our camper across the United States.

Psalm 104:23-NIV Then man goes out to his work, to his labor until evening.

Chapter 7
Getting Married

Joann and I both believe that God chose each of us for each other.

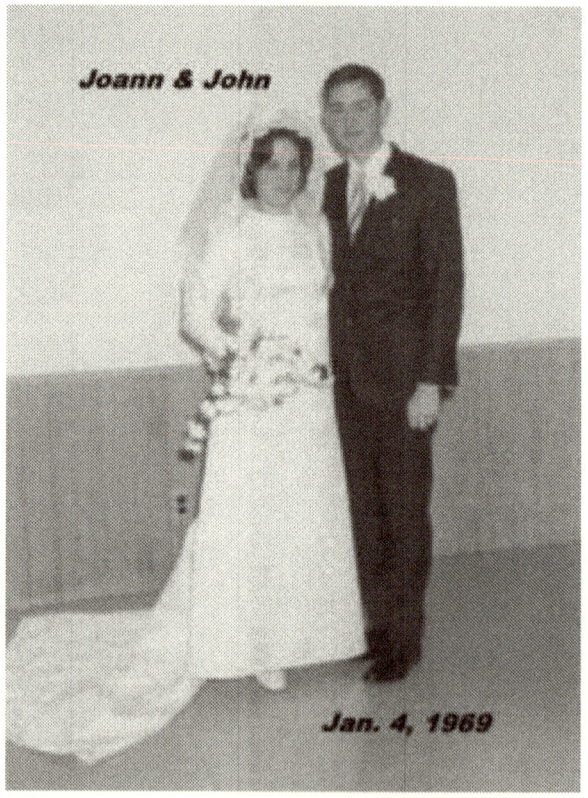

Joann & John

Jan. 4, 1969

"John Richard Bennett, do you take this woman to be your lawfully wedded wife"?

"Elizabeth Joann Barnett, do you take this man to be your lawfully wedded husband"? My father continued, "With the power vested in me..."

We can't believe this day has really arrived. Joann has had so much help planning this day; her mother, my mother, her grandmother, her maid of honor. We almost don't remember our engagement party any more. I had gotten up early that day and ridden my bicycle from East Marion to Riverhead, a distance of about twenty-five miles either way, to pick up our rings from Havils Jewelers. Being excited about the day, I had forgotten to take my insulin injection. The exercise kept me fine for several hours but my mind was wandering with the party that evening and I exacerbated the problem by not taking any tests. I was no longer taking pre supper insulin and everybody started arriving. We sat down and ate a great meal before I started getting sick to my stomach. Rationalizing about my heavy exercise and the excitement, I finally took my urine test and it was 4+ with positive ketones. I still didn't realize I'd forgotten to take my shot. My folks called the ambulance around 9PM and I spent several days in the hospital. Joann and I believe we came awfully close to not getting married.

But the day *was* finally here. Joann's niece, Toby, was the flower girl and she really stole the show. All the way down the aisle she was flirting with my oldest brother Jim who was part of the wedding party. The Ladies Aid Society of the church prepared our reception. Don't even remember what they served, but everyone said it was a great reception. It was January the 4th, 1969. We were originally going to get married on January the 1st but it was in the middle of the week, so we chose the first Saturday. The weather was gorgeous until the start of the reception—other than being cold. Then it started snowing - heavy! When we left the church there was at least six inches of snow on the ground and visibility was getting bad.

Our destination was the Radisson Inn, outside of Honesdale, Pa. We were to stay two nights before registering at Cove Haven Lodge on Lake Wallenpaupack. After four hours of driving I was getting blurry eyed from the snow and we finally stopped at a Howard Johnson just into New Jersey. We were only halfway to our destination. Calling the Radisson, they understood our predicament and cancelled our first night's reservation at no cost. There was two feet of new snow on the ground in the morning and five degrees below zero when I tried to start the car. Not even a ticking sound.

Finding and calling a local garage on a Sunday took nearly an hour. They brought and installed the new battery but the mechanic took interest in the 'Just Married' sign attached to the back of the car. He told me to go inside and stay warm while he finished and then he'd come in and give me the bill. Once I was back inside, he simply drove away. The clerk at the desk asked what had happened and once I explained he handed me our bill. It was imprinted with "Paid In Full". I had not given him any money.

Arriving at Cove Haven, we found that because of the 'blizzard' lots of folks, other than the skiers, had cancelled their reservations. Our room was upgraded at no extra cost. Electrically controlled drapes covered the whole front wall of floor to ceiling windows. We had a sunken bath, a large living room with fireplace, and an elevated bedroom area surrounded by a wrought iron railing accessible from the living room via three stairs. I remember being in my birthday suit peeking between the drapes waiting for them to deliver our breakfast in bed. When I told Joann our meal was coming she toggled the rheostat that controlled the drapes and they began to open. You've never seen anyone run across the living room, high jump the railing and get back in bed faster than I did. "Joann, I'll remember this".

Once Joann and I were married we moved into a mobile home in Riverhead, N.Y. Noel was born there and during her infancy I was still working shifts. One night after leaving for work around 11:15

PM for the midnight shift, I realized I had forgotten my keys to the mobile home. Going back home, all the lights were off. I assumed Joann had gone into our bedroom and retired. The door was locked and she didn't answer. That late at night I really didn't want to start hollering or knocking any louder. Our next door neighbor spoke to me through his window saying he was calling Joann on the phone. Finally getting into the mobile home, we had to recall the police to say there was no intruder. It was nice to know we had caring neighbors.

*   *   *

Leaving Pennsylvania in 1965, we moved to East Marion, Long Island. Just prior to getting my driver's permit (remember I had all sorts of problems getting insurance), I had asked Joann to go out with me to the Riverhead Raceway for the stock car races—our first real date. My brother was home at the time, so he offered to drive. My sister decided to go with us as well. Pulling into Joann's parent's driveway, we waited for several minutes until Joann's Mom came out to say hello. It seemed that Joann had seen my sister and wasn't going to come out, thinking I had a second girl with me. After finally leaving for the races, we *all* had a good time.

The following summer Joann's Dad hired me and the first job he assigned me was to paint the trim of the second story windows on his house. The first three windows I was to paint were above a porch. Setting the ladder next to a small unique fern, I began climbing the ladder but dropped the gallon of paint. It tipped upside down and landed directly on top of the fern. I found out Joann's Dad had searched for over a year to find her this particular fern. The fern died. I remember how horrible I felt seeing Joann's expression when she saw it. She married me anyway.

Whenever we go looking for plants I always look for this type of fern. After over thirty years of marriage I still haven't found one.

Ephesians 5:31-KJV For this cause shall a man leave his father and mother, and shall be joined unto his wife, and they two shall be one flesh.

Chapter 8
Kids

God's gift of children is an enormous blessing at the same time being an enormous responsibility.

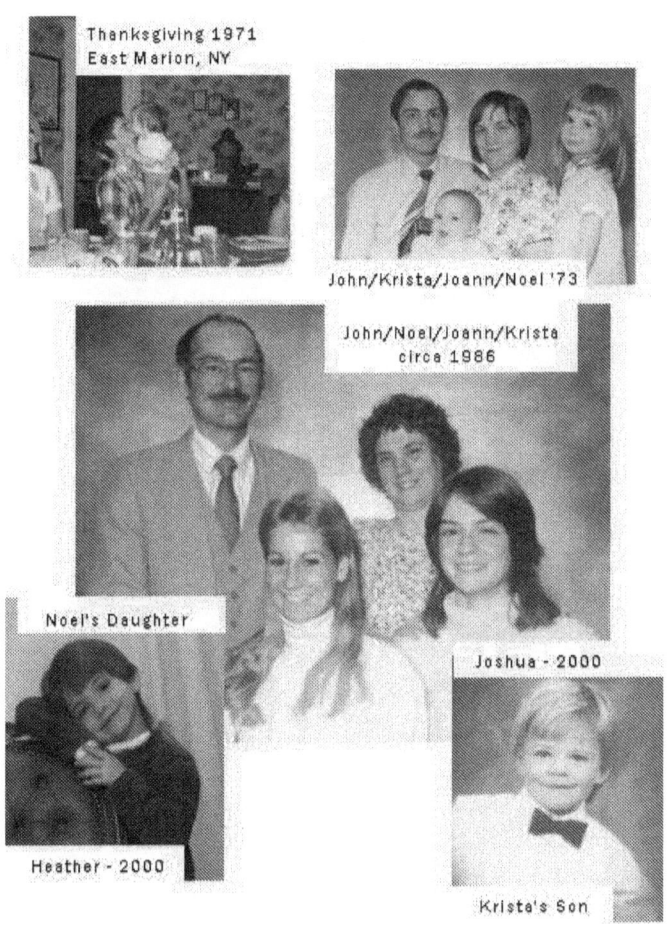

Thanksgiving 1971
East Marion, NY

John/Krista/Joann/Noel '73

John/Noel/Joann/Krista
circa 1986

Noel's Daughter

Joshua - 2000

Heather - 2000

Krista's Son

My wife, Joann, and I wanted children from the very first. However, we were apprehensive about the possiblity that any child of a diabetic has a tendency toward diabetes. We've studied all sorts of reports about genetic diabetes where the theory was that a generation is generally skipped before diabetes appears in offspring (now known to be false).

Other studies talk about diabetes being caused by childhood diseases - more recent studies even pointing to colds. DNA experiments have even isolated the 'diabetes' gene, although as yet, no one has been able to inhibit its generation.

Always being uninhibited with children, especially infants, I wanted a family as soon as possible. Our first daughter was born December 22, 1970. We brought her home on Christmas day, hence we named her Noel. She was our song of praise. Her middle name is Ruth after Joann's grandmother.

We celebrated with family a few days later. What occurred at my parents house is noteworthy. Invited for supper, we ate, opened presents, and had a beautiful family time together. It was dark when we started getting ready to go home. I went out to warm up the Corvair, returning to the house to start carrying presents to the car. On my last trip I had both arms full. I carried Noel in her carrier over one arm and a present in the other. Tempted to put the carrier on the car roof to open the door, I changed my mind and put the present there instead. Joann and I said our goodbyes, backed out of the driveway and headed home. In my rearview mirror I noticed an object come off the roof and start bouncing down the highway. Numerous times I've agonized over that object bouncing on the road possibly being Noel in her carrier. After pulling over to pick up the present, which was a 5" Sony TV that Joann could use in the kitchen, I only assumed it would be broken to pieces. Sony did a great job packing that box. There wasn't even a scratch on the TV and it worked for over six years.

Noel, as a baby, suffered from colic. My work hours really helped because I would get home shortly after midnight and handle baby duty so Joann could get some sleep before she went to work at 7AM. We had a rocking chair, which my grandfather had made by hand. It had been handed down to my mother, who handed it down to me. Rocking Noel was the only thing that put her to sleep at night. Many a night I would fall asleep with her on my shoulder in that chair.

At eleven months Noel decided to get up and walk, never having crawled. Joann and I were glad we were both young because we were both chasing around trying to keep up with our little girl. It got even more challenging when we found out our family was going to expand again and our mobile home wasn't going to be big enough. Buying a fix-me-up summer cottage in Sound Beach, I tested my construction ability. Soon, I had winterized the house and, eventually put on two extensions, digging out by hand the entire crawl space putting in a basement. Krista Louise was born in that house on July 11, 1973. Our little miss lucky (7-11).

During the latter months of Joann's pregnancy with Krista, when Joann could no longer bowl in our bowling league, I found a young man, Bob Lily, to fill in for her. The night of my highest game ever, Joann was not present. We bowled at the Rocky Point Bowling Alley and that night we were on lanes 15 & 16. Lane 16 was right next to the east wall. During my third game I rolled ten strikes in a row starting in frame one. Believing the eleventh ball to be a strike as well I was appalled to see the ten pin wobble but stay standing.

Normally a quiet, patient man and not knowing what caused my reaction, I turned to the wall and punched it with all my force. Breaking three metacarpal in my right hand, I was unable to finish the game. Bob drove my car to take me to the hospital. Can you imagine that Joann had no sympathy for me when I finally got home?

I never would have believed how different two sisters could be from each other. Both beautiful kids (yes I'm a little prejudiced), Noel

41

was the leader, Krista the follower. Noel being very loud, Krista being very quiet. Somewhere along the line, maybe when Noel was six and Krista four, we realized that disciplining either child took different strategies. With Noel, we first had to holler to get her attention, send her to her room until she got over being mad, then talk to her and explain how what she had done was wrong and how we expected her to react in the future. Trying this approach with Krista was a disaster. Krista has always tried to do exactly what her father and mother asked of her. When she did things wrong it was because she was following her sister's lead or just didn't know any better. One day I simply raised my voice to Krista in reprimand and she broke down in tears. From then on we only had to stop her from what she was doing and tell her not to do it again.

Both girls delighted us in so many ways. Shortly after Krista was born and both girls tested negative to diabetes, Joann and I decided 'not to push the odds' regarding a child with diabetes. I had an operation. We felt so proud of the girls and relieved they were both healthy.

Always being available to the kids was an absolute passion of mine. No matter what time of day or night, they were comfortable enough to pull me aside and speak what was on their mind or discuss what had happened during their day. Even when subjects got really personal and Joann got embarassed by some of the questions, Dad would simply give the best advice he was capable of. The "no hesitation, no condescension" attitude paid off high dividends in later years. If either of the girls had had a hard time it was Dad's lap they curled up into. Years later, after each of the girls had a small infant of their own (of course separate occasions separated by years), I was called in the wee hours of the morning because they couldn't quiet down the baby. Arriving at the house, it was only minutes before my grandchild would calm down and go to sleep on my shoulder. On her respective occasion Noel turned and lovingly said to me, "Dad I hate you".

Lack of good diabetes control can cause all sorts of emotional instability. When I occasionally had a high blood sugar I found I was out of sorts, even testy. Being there for my wife and kids was always one *BIG* incentive to keep under the best possible control I was capable of.

Krista was attending Vacation Bible School (VBS) one summer at Sound Beach Community Church where we were members. The Pastor asked the kids if there was anyone whose father would be able to bring a real live sheep for a special function during VBS. Krista immediately raised her hand and said, "My Dad can get anything!" What a spot I was in. No way was I going to let my daughter down if I didn't have to, but where in the world was I going to get a sheep. Telling my story to a friend at work, Karl Abrams responded by telling me his father-in-law raised sheep. There was a very happy little girl and a very surprised Pastor the day I drove up with sheep in my truck.

Matthew 18:2-6-NIV He called a little child and had him stand among them. And he said: "I tell you the truth, unless you change and become like little children, you will never enter the kingdom of heaven. Therefore, whoever humbles himself like this child is the greatest in the kingdom of heaven. And whoever welcomes a little child like this in my name welcomes me. But if anyone causes one of these little ones who believe in me to sin, it would be better for him to have a large millstone hung around his neck and to be drowned in the depths of the sea."

Chapter 9
Diabetic Retinopathy

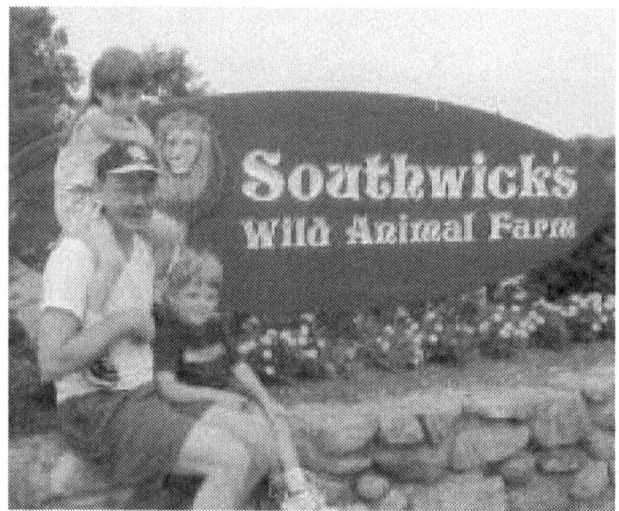

Heather, Papa, Joshua 2000

While on vacation one week, I was raking leaves on a neighbor's lawn. Needing to remove leaves from a bush, I leaned into the bush to grasp them and a twig went into my eye. Going home to wash out my eye, I noticed what I thought was a slice on the cornea. Calling my doctor I was referred to an optometrist. I immediately called the optometrist and was informed that he just had a cancellation for 11:00AM, an hour from now, and if I could get there he would see me. During my examination he diagnosed a small laceration of the cornea and prescribed an ointment to assist in the healing process. He also blew my mind when he asked how long I had been a diabetic.

Continuing, he explained that I had second stage diabetic retinopathy, which is a proliferation of blood vessels in the retina and that I would require laser treatments to cauterize these proliferations.

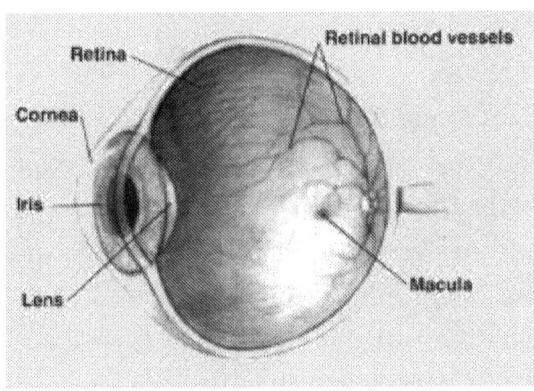

After he referred me to Suffolk Ophthalmology he called Dr. Charles Beyrer, his friend and ophthalmologist who worked there. If I could be there in an hour he would see me that day. Dr. Beyrer advised I have someone with me to drive me home after the examination. His reaffirming the optometrist's diagnosis came as no surprise, however, his saying that there had been a cancellation for a treatment the following morning at 9:00AM did.

My vehicle at the time was an old clunker of a pickup truck. Joann ended up driving me home in rush hour traffic and really had a bad time. She was nervous simply with my eye problem; her nervousness now being complicated by the traffic and my truck. Finally arriving home she was frantic! She just couldn't face getting behind the wheel again in the morning. I agreed. If worse came to worse, I'd simply drive myself then sit in the waiting room after my treatment until my eyes were no longer dilated and drive myself home.

At 5:00AM the next morning our Pastor called.

"Something woke me up early this morning. There's some reason I felt I had to call you this early. What's happening? What can I do for you?"

Not having spoken to the pastor since Sunday he had no way of knowing I needed a ride.

After our pastor drove Joann and I to my appointment, I had drops applied to my eyes to get them dilated. An hour or so later they asked me to go to the treatment room. Dr. Beyrer explained the laser treatment, positioned me in front of the hardware and began to work on my left eye. It's difficult to describe the feeling of a laser beam as it enters your eye. Your pupil is fully dilated and your eyelids are held open with the insertion of the lens of the laser 'gun'. I declined the option of being strapped into the device framing my head and specially designed to rest my chin. I compare the discomfort to someone holding a thumbtack to your eye and every few seconds applying extra pressure. Two hours and several hundred lasers later my eye was patched, another appointment was scheduled and I was allowed to go home. My thinking I would have been able to drive myself home was a real joke.

My headache lasted until well into the evening. Because my head had to be elevated, I slept in my recliner. Saturday and Sunday gave me two days of rest before going back to work on Monday. Because my vision was impaired, they put me on restricted duty and used me to train new computer operators. This included hands-on loading of paper into printers and loading magnetic tapes into tape drives. It was amazing what I could do from memory.

Later that week, Suffolk Ophthalmology contacted me. Dr. Beyer had been impressed by my demeanor during the first treatment and asked me if I would be willing to talk to other ophthalmologists who were being taught laser technology while I was undergoing treatments. Because I was willing, I never paid a cent for the following six treatments. Joann and I were even treated to buffet dinners.

Having also purchased a new pickup after the first treatment, Joann no longer had a problem driving me to my appointments.

If you look in the glossary under retinopathy you will see the words poorly controlled diabetes. Questioning endocrinologists, three out of four agree with this definition. However, the fourth believes that even with "decent" control, long term diabetes can and sometimes does cause problems such as retinopathy. Agreeing with this approach doesn't make me feel any better that I still required laser treatments for retinopathy.

I had diabetes twenty-four years before beginning laser treatments. I had prided myself on good diabetic control, doing everything possible at the time to stay within proper guidelines. During these twenty-four years I was under the care of a General Practitioner. During my earlier diabetic life, endocrinologists were not readily available. Today, an endocrinologist is a most valuable asset while attempting to achieve the best control of diabetes.

Today it's necessary to wear one pair of glasses to read, another pair for driving, yet another for computer work. It doesn't seem a big compromise after being legally blind for six months. My eyesight didn't get worse because of the retinopathy. The laser treatments actually saved my sight. Only aging has caused me to need glasses.

My laser treatments (pan retinal photocoagulation) started with the argon laser which emits a blue light. Its predecessor was the ruby laser; its descendants were the carbon dioxide laser and neodymium YAG laser.

My advice to any diabetic:

♦ have an ophthalmologist examine yours eyes twice a year
♦ become a member of your own health-care team
♦ beyond your primary health care provider, work with an endocrinologist

Becoming friends with my ophthalmologist and his entire staff, I have an entire collection of pictures of my retina during my fluorescein scans as well as before and after photocoagulation. My scrapbooks, plural, are full of articles about the first laser treatments and the progression of different styles of lasers as well as a collection of personal diabetes paraphernalia.

Some may say everything that happened, from the time I lacerated my cornea to the completion of my laser treatments was pure happenstance; others will attribute it to sheer luck. No one will convince me that there wasn't divine intervention in how everything worked out the way it did.

Deuteronomy 4:9a-NIV Only be careful, and watch yourselves closely so that you do not forget the things your eyes have seen or let them slip from your heart as long as you live.

Chapter 10
Daughter Diagnosed Type-I

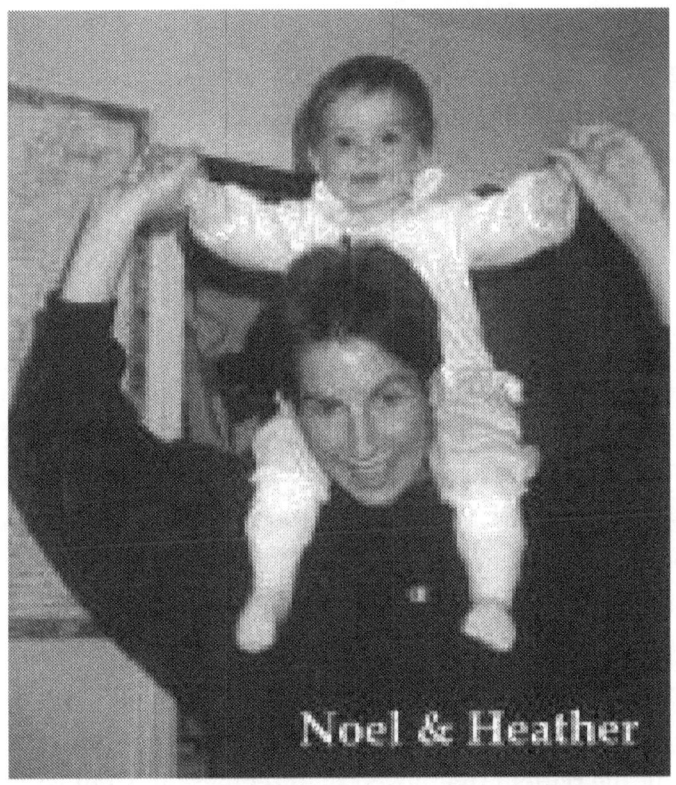

Noel & Heather

Once a year Joann and I would have each girl tested for diabetes and I was refilled with relief each time the tests came back negative.

This relief lasted until Noel was sixteen when she was diagnosed with diabetes. Recognizing the signs and getting affirmation from high blood sugar tests and then a glucose tolerance test, she was admitted into Stony Brook Hospital to learn about her disease. This really took me back in time. Going to the hospital after work the first day she was admitted, I remember walking into her room where a nurse was attempting to teach her how to give her own injection. She was making a fuss and I heard, "My Dad is the only one who is going to teach me how to take insulin". It was great for my ego but not very practical.

Being a teenager new to diabetes is so much more difficult than my getting used to diabetes at the age of six. All my habits were formed around diabetes. Noel had to *change* all her habits. No more sweets with school pals any time you wanted them; no skipping meals when you weren't hungry. Now you had to take insulin injections every day. There were also some good differences compared to years ago, however. One is, people with diabetes no longer have to weigh foods on a gram scale. Instead, Noel learned food exchanges.

My own training on food exchanges had come several years before Noel was diagnosed. At the same time Noel started taking blood sugar readings, I replaced my Clinitest Kit with the same self-test blood-glucose monitor she was given. What an advance in diabetes care. No more four-hour-ago sugar results. Actual current blood sugar results took less than thirty seconds. Breakthroughs in diabetes research are becoming more apparent all the time.

Now I know what my mother had gone through. It's so much easier being the patient diagnosed than the parent. I felt so helpless. In this case, my number one priority had to be supporting my daughter. Comparing my mother's experience to mine, however, I realize that my situation was much easier than hers. She had to learn everything at the same time I did. In Noel's case, her father and mother had already lived with a diabetic patient for years.

There were so many differences between my embracing and accepting the 'world' of diabetes and Noel's hesitation and reluctance. She was afraid to tell anyone about her disease. She would not cope with a new situation until forced to, going through mood swings before coming to grips with the changes her condition brought into her life.

Yet Noel always had more strength than even she realized. After she got married, she and her husband decided to have a baby. Being a brittle diabetic, one who can rapidly go from a low blood sugar to a high blood sugar and vice versa, Noel went to a doctor specializing in maternal diabetes. The last month of her pregnancy she was resident in the hospital. Once Heather was born, Noel was told that, because of the complications of this delivery, she should not become pregnant again.

Heather Elizabeth Stewart was born on August 31st, 1996. Elizabeth must be a good name. It's my mother's first name, it's Joann's mother's first name, it's Joann's actual first name, now Heather's middle name. Of course, before the first week of Heather's life was over she had Papa wrapped around her tiny little finger.

A year or so later, Noel's sister Krista presented her husband with a strapping baby boy, Joshua Louis Carlino. Louis is Joann's Dad's first name.

Last year (2000), Noel's endocrinologist recommended that she go on the insulin pump and suggested the newest model from MiniMed, the 508. Before making her decision, of course, she had to confer with Dad. Not only did she convince me that she needed the pump, she convinced me that I needed one as well. Speaking with my endocrinologist, she saw no reason why I shouldn't be on the pump, so I got one too. Endocrinologists have their own Diabetes Educator who train patients on pump use. Noel was connected to her pump one week to the day before I was.

*   *   *

51

For as long as I can remember a snowstorm meant snow blowing. While living in Sound Beach, New York, I cleared over a dozen driveways after each storm. One homeowner was a very special lady to my wife and me. Her name was Ruth Jensen, a Norwegian woman with heavy accent and a simply loving lady. She absolutely adored both Noel and Krista.

At age seventy-eight, she had been widowed for many years, living on her husbands pension and social security. Ruth attended church where my family and I attended. She asked me one day if I knew someone who could do her driveway. Explaining she couldn't afford much, in lieu of monetary payment, her work would be done just before lunch so she could serve Joann and me a meal before I continued my rounds. We found she would listen to weather reports diligently and prior to a snowstorm would stock up on certain cooking items. Ruth lifted her phone off the hook each morning of a storm so nobody could disturb her. She would not only make lunch, but we always left with a large cookie tin of "krumkake". These light crisp cone shaped delights were worth dying for.

For seven years I was spoiled and loved in this manner before Mrs. Jensen was placed in a Nursing Home and then passed away. I praise the Lord that some day, either upon His return or during my life after death, as promised in Scripture, I will see her again.

Genesis 29:16-NIV Now Laban had two daughters; the name of the older was Leah, and the name of the younger was Rachel.

Chapter 11
Insulin Pump

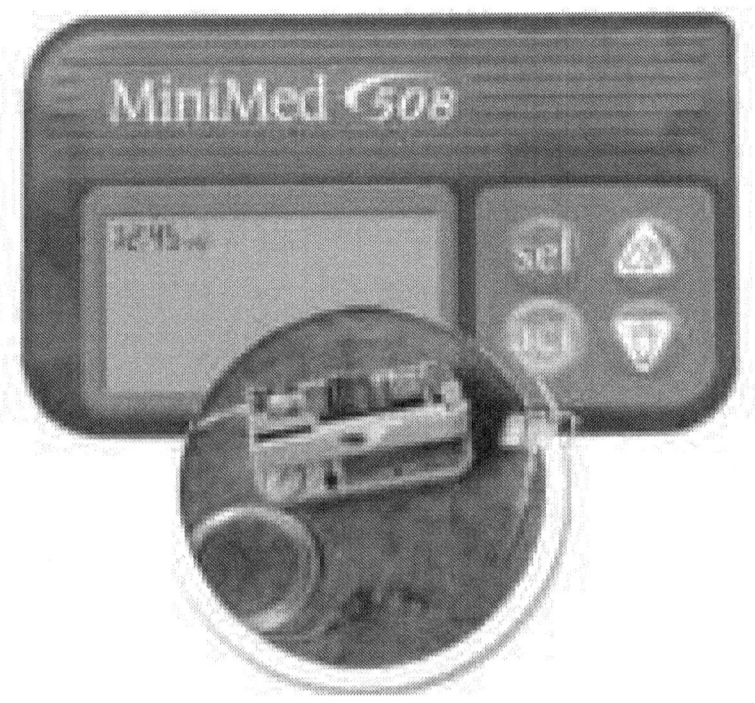

    I had watched with interest the diabetes magazine articles about insulin pump therapy for several years, but with three—sometimes four—insulin injections a day, I thought a pump would be a luxury rather than a necessity.

    My endocrinologist thought that I would be an excellent candidate for the pump. When we discovered my insurance policy would cover the pump in full, I proceeded to order the MiniMed 508 as per her recommendation. Within two weeks I had received my pump and supplies but I had to await training. Previously scheduling a week's vacation, my training by the Diabetes Educator and RN Dorothy Stevens would have to wait another week. Dorothy and I hit it off on our first introduction. The training went smoothly and when connecting my pump for the first time I went directly to insulin. Noel, on the other hand, had had her training the previous week but she was to practice with the pump using saline solution instead of insulin. Within a few days, she had graduated to Humalog.

This is the first time I had used Humulin insulin. It was recommended that I use Humalog in my new pump. The supplies that came with the pump consisted of alcohol swabs, IV Preps, a Sof-set inserter, reservoirs, and 24-inch quick release Sof-set Micro infusion set. It may sound complicated at first, but within a week I had it mastered. Now instead of *multiple insulin injections every day,* I am *only* required to change my Sof-set insertion site *once every two to three days.*

Wearing the pump just under a year, I've gained an even lower A1C (glycosolated hemoglobin) test without the extreme highs and lows I had been getting. Noel's test differences were even more remarkable than mine. We were now receiving a constant supply of insulin around the clock. This is considered a *basal rate.* During certain times of the day a diabetic may require different amounts of insulin to keep a stable blood sugar reading. The insulin pump allows the programming of multiple (more than I'll ever need) basal rates. Between two o'clock and six o'clock in the morning, I need three-tenths of a unit less insulin per hour than at any other time during the day. After I've eaten the first time during the day, my basal rate needs to be increased for two hours by two-tenths of a unit per hour. Currently, I have seven different basal settings per twenty-four hour period. The pump also has a separate set of alternate basal rate settings. These allow me to modify basal rates for a short time period without modifying standard basal rates. When I have a cold, I require more insulin. During this period, I set my alternate basal rate settings two-tenths of a unit per hour higher than my standard rate.

With basal rate(s) set so that I have a consistent blood-glucose reading throughout the day, I then need to take into consideration my exercise and diet. With exercise, I can either take less insulin or eat more carbohydrate. Being a good eater my preference is extra food. On occasion, however, the quick-release infusion set has allowed me to actually disconnect from the pump without removing the infusion set. I have disconnected during periods of heavy exercise, but most often only to bathe or shower. My current pump is not waterproof and cannot get wet. When I kayak, I have an accessory that is waterproof that shelters the pump within a clear plastic shell with a soft watertight opening for the tubing to pass through.

Diet requires carb counting and an additional infusion of insulin, the *bolus*. All food packages contain the number of grams of carbohydrate per serving. To calculate my bolus, I multiply the grams of carbohydrate per serving by the number of servings I am eating, then divide that number by the number of carbohydrate that one unit of insulin takes care of for me. This number was defaulted when I first received my pump and then derived by experimenting with how much insulin was required to balance my blood sugar with a known quantity of intake. First starting on my pump, this number was eleven(11). Within two days I knew my body needed one(1) unit of insulin for every thirteen(13) grams of carbohydrate.

Here's an example: I intend to eat an egg salad sandwich and a glass of ice tea for lunch. Note - All carbohydrate values are fictitious! They are only used here for ease of calculation.

	serving size	carbs/ serving	# of servings
bread	1 slice	24	2
egg	1	4	2
light mayonnaise	1 tspn.	9	1
diet ice tea	8 oz.	0	

(24 * 2) + (4 * 2) + (9 * 1) = 65 / 13 = 5.0
My bolus for lunch is 5.0 units.

Now I know both "exchanges" and "carb counting".

Almost all fast food restaurants have lists of carbohydrates for all their specials. I don't advocate extensive eating at these types of places, but it's nice to go out with the grand-kids once in a while and be able to calculate the amount of insulin you need to handle the meal you're eating.

During the year I've been on my pump, I have come to realize that blood-glucose testing is even more important than when I was injecting insulin. We don't need to discuss low blood sugars that always have symptoms that are readable to a diabetic, but instead talk about the possibilty of high sugars, which are less discernible. Lengthy periods of disconnecting from the pump are dangerous. Even after heavy exercise I find my sugars starting to rise again within an hour unless I've reconnected. Unless I test on a frequent and regular basis, I would be less likely to recognize a high blood sugar until it was much higher than I would want it to be. There have also been times, especially on weekends, when my schedule is different than during the week, that I have forgotten to take a bolus. Within thirty minutes of ingesting food my blood sugars are already dramatically rising. Without testing, this can become extremely dangerous.

My personal schedule of testing is as follows:

- before breakfast (8AM)
- before lunch (noon)
- before supper (5PM)
- before bed (10PM)
- before driving (at least twice a day)
- upon arising (4-5AM)
- when I feel myself going low

Noel and I both enjoy attending an 'Insulin Pumpers' group. Just like Camp Joslin brings boys with diabetes together to learn and share their experiences, the pumper groups bring together fellow insulin pumpers. We learn of new pumps, new blood glucose testing devices, advances in diabetes research and discuss things like different insurance companies or how to be prepared for traveling, etc. Our group has a great bunch of pumpers and is led by my Diabetes Educator Dorothy Stevens.

Note: MiniMed, the maker of my pump, has recently become MedTronic MiniMed.

Romans 6:13-KJV Neither yield ye your members as instruments of unrighteousness unto sin: but yield yourselves unto God, as those that are alive from the dead, and your members as instruments of righteousness unto God.

Chapter 12
Blood Glucose Monitor

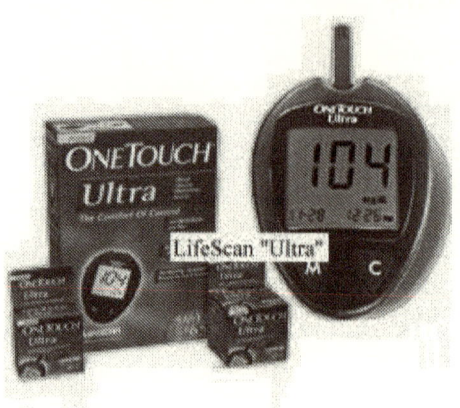

LifeScan "Ultra"

There's a night and day difference between using a blood glucose monitor and the old method of urine tests with a Clinitest kit.

Prior to blood glucose monitoring I would test my urine to see if I was passing sugar. If so, it would mean my blood glucose level was higher than it should be. The body is an amazing 'computer'. When a person's blood sugar level gets to a certain level, the brain tells the pancreas to secrete enough insulin to handle the sugar or glucose or glycogen. Once the lower boundary is reached the brain tells the pancreas to stop its insulin secretion. For a diabetic, the brain is telling the pancreas to secrete insulin but the pancreas just can't do it. This is diabetes mellitus in very simple laymen terms. The insulin allows the body to use the glucose properly. Without insulin the blood stream contains this unused glucose and the body attempts to get rid of it. By means of two other organs, the liver and kidneys, this glucose is filtered and finally passed out of the body. Prolonged high blood glucose causes a strain on these organs as well as contributing to other complications such as retinopathy.

For years I tested urine to find out how my control was. Because urine is a body waste the test results are delinquent by up to four hours. When there is no other means for testing you put up with what you have. Because there was nothing else, Clinitest was great. If the result was negative you were not passing any sugar in the urine. Tests could range from negative to 4+, each giving a different color that could be compared to a color chart. If I was 4+ I also tested for ketones. If ketones were present my doctor would normally send me for a fasting blood sugar. Every few months I would have blood sugars that would test how much glucose was being 'retained' by the blood stream rather than being properly used by the body. There is a test called an A1C or HbA1C or glycosylated hemoglobin that counts how much glucose has remained unused in the blood stream within the last three or four months. The ratio standards for an insulin dependent diabetic with a good A1C is now 6.5 or less.

Several years ago I was introduced to a self-glucose-monitoring kit. Finding several articles about them on the internet I requested a referral from my endocrinologist. She vouched for several companies and I selected LifeScan. My first monitor was the "OneTouch Profile". Using a small drop of blood obtained from the fingertips an accurate blood glucose level result would be reported in forty-five seconds. These blood sugar levels are current and they appear in a digital readout. While I was still injecting insulin I would be able to determine the amount of insulin to inject to obtain my desired blood sugar level. Now that I'm using an insulin pump, I believe taking frequent blood sugars is even more important. When first starting pump therapy I wanted to know what my best basal rate was for any given time period. Splitting twenty-four hours into four hour chunks, I tested every hour within a chunk for a week to determine what my best possible basal rate (remember basal rates and boluses from previous chapter) was for that particular chunk of time. I now have seven different basal rates within each twenty-four hour period. Tests prior to meals allow me to do simple arithmetic to determine how much insulin to take for my bolus. Without the monitor these adjustments would be impossible to make.

Nearly a year passed before I started using LifeScan's new "FastTake" meter. Smaller than the "Profile" and packaged in a small case with velcro straps to fasten the kit onto my belt I was now able to get results within fifteen seconds. The kit contained the meter, a lancet device, a bottle of twenty-five test strips, a supply of lancets and a control agent used to verify accuracy. Now everything was on my person. Not only that, but I don't even look out of place. Nearly everyone is carrying a cellphone on their belts now. I've simple exchanged an insulin pump and a meter for the cellphone.

Just recently I obtained LifeScan's latest and greatest, the "OneTouch Ultra" (see photo above). My test results are now reported in five seconds. I'm actually getting spoiled. The "Ultra" has the capability of using different sites for obtaining the blood sample as well. Now instead of just the fingertips, you can use your forearms. However, I would be remiss if I didn't mention that a recent article by the American Diabetes Association (ADA) suggests that persons using an insulin pump not use alternate site testing. Fingertip testing is still the most accurate.

For those of us who have used these meters for quite some time, there are products available to help keep the fingertips soft and supple. I personally use an aloe-vera product called "Fingers" by MedTronic MiniMed.

Romans 12:1,2 KJV I beseech you therefore, brethren, by the mercies of God, that ye present your bodies a living sacrifice, holy, acceptable unto God, which is your reasonable service. And be not conformed to this world: but be ye transformed by the renewing of your mind, that ye may prove what is that good, and acceptable, and perfect, will of God.

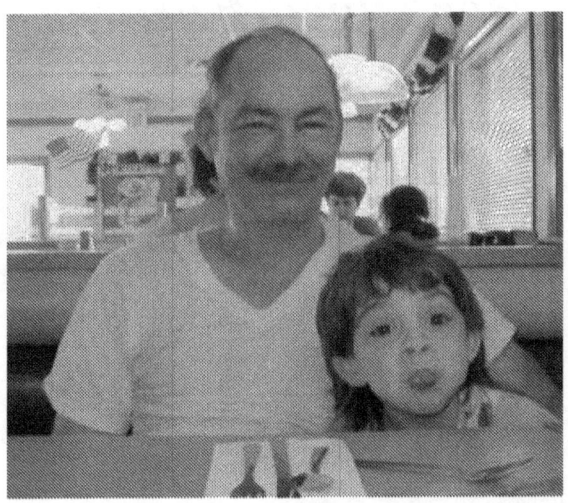

Chapter 13
Perceived Futures

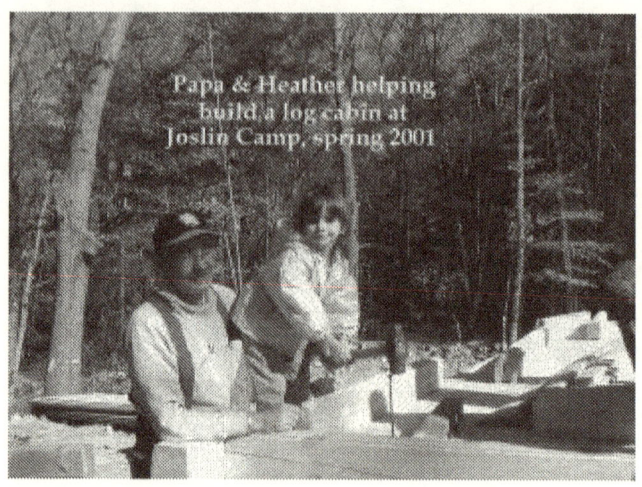

Papa & Heather helping build a log cabin at Joslin Camp, spring 2001

I had expected a cure for diabetes within my lifetime. Now I pray it happens within my daughter's lifetime.

Newly diagnosed diabetics can't comprehend the advantages in diabetic research and management compared to fifty years ago. Few current diabetics have ever used a clinitest kit. Instead, self-blood-glucose monitors are the norm. Insulin has changed dramatically from my old U40 NPH to today's Humulin Humalog.

When I was a youngster at camp (1957), I was chosen with five other campers to go to the Joslin Clinic in Boston to be a guinea pig for a new oral insulin, "orinase". None of the Type-I diabetics would be able to use this tablet, although it made a remarkable inroad for Type-II diabetes. There have been numerous advances in the range of oral insulins, which now have reached the market.

The agent we used to use to combat hypoglycemia was raw coke syrup. When it got hot during the summer months it was the most horrid tasting sickeningly sweet viscous liquid you ever tasted. Today, there are all sorts of choices according to preference. There are gels and syrups in single wrapped foil sleeves, but my favorite is glucose tablets. Purchased in ten(10) tablet water-resistant tubes, each tablet is four(4) grams of carbohydrate, in all sorts of different flavors. I like these because they are solid, can be easily extracted from their dispensers and, regardless of the temperature, always taste the same.

Syringes are now mainly used once and then thrown away. They can be obtained in numerous sizes from full CC to pre-drawn 1/4 CC. The actual needle gauge is minuscule compared to original needles.

Insulin pumps started out nearly the size of a business envelope and weighed over a pound. The newer pumps can fit into the palm of your hand and weigh less than six ounces. The newest MedTronic MiniMed pump, the "Paradigm", although not yet available for purchase, is even waterproof for 30 seconds up to 10 feet.

Self-blood-glucose monitors no longer take 30 seconds to get a result. Newer models use less of a blood sample and take less time, yet have still become more accurate. There are models now available that use alternate test sites than the fingers, although these are not recommended for pump users. My new "LifeScan Ultra" meter replaces its big brother, the "FastTake" meter. It uses less of a blood sample, is not as sensitive to heat or cold and reports the result in five seconds.

Years ago, there was no way to stop or even slow down proliferating blood vessels in the retina. Once they burst into the eye's vitreous fluid, a patient is literally blind. Today, laser therapy is making astronomical strides in treating diabetic retinopathy. I had laser treatments two decades ago. Frequent eye examinations show no subsequent problems with my retinas.

DNA testing, DCCT Trials and islet cell transplant articles are appearing more and more often. Pancreas transplants combined with kidney transplants have proven to be much more effective for a diabetic than having one or the other transplanted by itself. Transplants are becoming more common. Rather than having to have multiple insulin injections a transplant patient is only required to take an oral immunosuppressant, which is necessary for all who receive a transplant of any kind.

Giant steps are being taken each year towards a cure for diabetes mellitus. Without being a soothsayer or prophet, I'm going to step out on a limb and make a prediction. I do not believe Type-II diabetes will ever be cured. Instead, I believe that Type-I diabetes will be cured and that Type-II diabetes will simply disappear. I offer no time frame, however.

Within the next decade I can envision an implanted blood glucose monitor that will be readable by the patient whenever he or she wishes. There even may be a pump without the need of an infusion set. I have been taking notes for this book for quite some time and they refer to the possibility of taking fingertip blood samples without the necessity of using a lancette. I recently sent my diabetes educator a reference to just such a device that uses a hand held laser device.

Many years ago I went to an Oral Roberts Crusade to ask for the "faith healing" of my diabetes. You've read this book so you know it didn't happen. I believe in a faith that could have done just that. However, there were different plans for my life. I am convinced that God wanted me to live with an infirmity to ease others who are having difficulty living with that same infirmity. Being there for my daughter is a prime example. Also, I'm hoping this book will help you or someone you know to deal with diabetes. Hopefully you'll learn from my mistakes and come to realize even to a greater degree than I have, how full and rich life can be with diabetes.

May God bless!

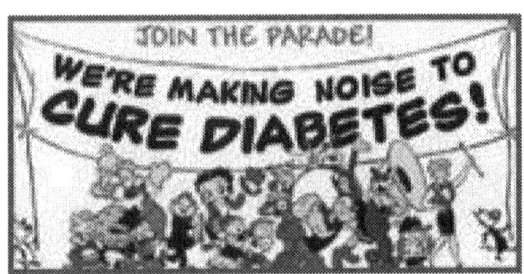

Romans 8:38,39-KJV For I am persuaded, that neither death, nor life, nor angels, nor principalities, nor powers, nor things present, nor things to come, Nor height, nor depth, nor any other creature, shall be able to separate us from the love of God, which is in Christ Jesus our Lord.

John R. Bennett

Testimonials

I had the pleasure and the privilege of meeting John Bennett on August 3, 2000. He had decided to change his method of treating his Diabetes from multiple daily injections to using an Insulin Pump. I found John to be a very disciplined, organized person who was very knowledgeable about Diabetes and truly tried to have the very best control. He was eager to learn all that he could about this new way of treating Diabetes, however I think that he had his doubts as to whether he could improve on what he felt was good control. It wasn't long when he called me and said," I no longer have the lows that were causing me so much trouble." His Insulin Pump improved John's world. John never complained about his world as a person with Diabetes and he has a very active lifestyle. He never let Diabetes restrict his activities. He is an avid kayaker, loves the outdoors, and gives freely of his time to help others. His volunteer work at Joslin Camp is very close to his heart. He has told me about his time at Joslin as a youngster and although he has fond memories, he wants to make it better for other children living with Diabetes. I felt very fortunate to be the educator to assist him with his Insulin Pump training.

John also extended himself when he learned that I coordinate a support group for pump patients in our practice. He has established a web page for our group, northshorepumpers.com as a service to our patients. It has meant a great deal to new patients who are contemplating pump therapy. John's upbeat, positive attitude has seen him through some difficult times. John's cup is never half empty, it is always half full.

Dorothy E. Stevens, R.N. & Diabetes Educator

I have known John Bennett for over twenty years. Like most people, I had a general knowledge of diabetes but never actually knew someone suffering with the disease. Over the years as I got to know John better, I learned that there are two types of diabetes. One that requires insulin and usually starts at an early age and the other non-insulin dependent type that is the more common form and shows up in adulthood. John has the insulin dependent or juvenile onset type.

It wasn't an uncommon sight to see John checking his blood sugar level and giving himself an injection. He was always very diligent with his injections, exercise, and diet. He knew the portions of food he could safely eat and lead a vigorous and active life style. If you didn't know him, you would never have suspected that he had diabetes.

John is also a man with a tremendous work ethic. Occasionally, his work ethic would get in the way of his insulin injections and hypoglycemia would result. It was a scary situation to witness but quickly overcome with the ingestion of a little sugar.

Diabetes has many side effects. One of the most serious effects the capillaries in the back of the eye. On at least two occasions, John underwent laser eye surgeries to correct this condition.

A deeply spiritual man, John has always been upbeat about his condition. He is also very pro-active in helping others learn and cope with the disease. He regularly volunteers his time in the summer at the Joslin Camp in Massachusetts to help others learn how to regulate their diabetes.

Paul Kessler
Section Head for Distributed Systems
Brookhaven National Laboratory (Retired)

"My views of John Bennett and his Diabetes"

In thinking about how to describe "John Bennett and his diabetes", it immediately became clear to me that this is not really about the diabetes...it's about the person. In all the years I've known John, he never really has emphasized the diabetes and never complained about it. Diabetes never dominates the conversation, never is mentioned as a hardship, never used as an excuse for avoiding something. The only memory that I have of John talking about diabetes, relative to himself, is a positive statement he made—many years ago—that having diabetes actually gave him an advantage over other people! If I'm remembering correctly, John felt that he grew up understanding a lot more about food and nutrition than the ordinary person did! In learning to deal with his condition he also recognized and capitalized on the importance of physical exercise...and that aspect has always been important in carrying out his daily life.

John is one of the most energetic, enthusiastic, motivated people that I've ever known. This relates to his professional career as well as his personal life. At work, he requires and thrives on work overload, feeding on multiple project assignments in order to feel truly satisfied. Being asked to work unusual hours, late or early, was never a problem (although he easily could have used diabetes as an excuse). Outside of work, he's always been moving in many directions at once—whether it's helping his family dig out a basement; working on a church project; cutting down trees full of ants with a power saw; plowing snow off driveways; driving to jury duty in Brooklyn from Long Island in a snow storm; cycling through mountains; racing his kayak; and the list goes on and on. Where does the diabetes enter in? When does he even have time to take/check his insulin? I have no idea, but again, this is not a major "bulletin" in John's life.

This is not to say that he doesn't understand the seriousness and potential complications of diabetes. He certainly does...and has had his share of problems, such as the visual complications of diabetic retinopathy. But even through that serious situation, after undergoing laser treatments that would have taken most people out of their normal life patterns for weeks (if not longer), John was back at work in record time. He dealt with the problem, and moved ahead, unconsciously setting a great example, becoming a true role for others that might be in a similar situation. The only time that diabetes gets a direct spotlight from John, is when he's working in support of a specific event—whether it's volunteering to speak at a Diabetic camp, raising funds via a physical event (such as miles of walking, cycling, kayaking), or just talking informally to kids or other groups about his life experience with diabetes.

I remember giving a speech once, at a luncheon celebration of John's 25 years (or so) at BNL, and describing him (using the Shakespeare line) as a person whose "candle" not only "burns at both ends", but also in the middle. Think about this analogy...it gives a really bright light...in all directions...but in his case, in spite of all the flame, it doesn't look like its about to burn out for quite some time.

S. Sevian - Manager of Self Assessment &
Quality Assurance
Brookhaven National Laboratory

Glossary

Unless otherwise noted, words and terms from MEDLINEplus http://www.nlm.nih.gov/medlineplus/dictionaries.html a web version of "U.S. National Library of Medicine (NLM), 8600 Rockville Pike, Bethesda, MD 20894".

Other sources:

By permission, From Merriam-Webster's Collegiate® Dictionary at www.Merriam-Webster.com, ©2001 by Merriam-Webster, Incorporated.

By permission, From Michael Bliss's The Discovery of Insulin (Chicago: University of Chicago Press, 1982).

*   *   *

A1C - see Hb A1C

blood-glucose level

Most dietary carbohydrate eventually ends up as glucose in the blood. Excess glucose is converted to glycogen for storage by the liver and skeletal muscles after meals. Glycogen is gradually broken down to glucose and released into the blood by the liver between meals. Excess glucose is converted to triglyceride for energy storage.

Glucose is a major source of energy for most cells of the body. Some cells (for example, brain and red blood cells), are almost totally dependent on blood glucose as a source of energy. The brain, in fact, requires that glucose concentrations in the blood remain within a certain range in order to function normally. Concentrations less than about 30 milligrams per deciliter (mg/dl) or greater than about 300 mg/dl can produce confusion or unconsciousness.

blood-glucose monitor

Blood sugar testing, also called "self-monitoring," is done using a special meter called a glucometer to check the amount of glucose in a drop of blood. Testing is usually done before meals and at bedtime, though more frequent testing may be needed during times of illness or stress. If it is done on a regular basis, testing informs the diabetic patient and their healthcare provider how well diet, exercise, and medication are working together to control their diabetes.

carbohydrate

The primary function of carbohydrates is to provide energy for the body, especially the brain and the nervous system. The body breaks down starches and sugars into a substance called glucose, which is used for energy by the body.

It is recommended that somewhere between 40 to 60% of our total calories come from carbohydrates, preferably from complex carbohydrates (starches) and naturally occurring sugars rather than processed or refined sugars.

High-sugar foods are simple carbohydrates that provide calories, but minimal nutritional benefits.

On the other hand, complex carbohydrates provide calories, vitamins and minerals as well as fiber. Therefore, it is wise to limit processed and refined sugars.

clinitest

A screening test to detect the presence of various substances in the urine that chemically react with an indicator metallic dye (cupric sulfate). The most common reducing substances examined include glucose or galactose.

If the Clinitest tablet turns blue, this indicates the present of a urinary reducing substance such as glucose (as seen in diabetes). A simple urine dipstick test that is specific for glucose can be performed.

If the dipstick test is positive, then you have a high level of glucose in the blood, and the glucose is spilling over into the urine.

conventional control

Diabetes results from deficient insulin or insensitivity to insulin. Type I diabetics require daily injections of insulin. Injection of too much or too little insulin can be dangerous.

Normal values: 64 to 126 mg/dl

Note: mg/dl = milligrams per deciliter.

dawn phenomenon [MEDLINEplus - On-line Medical Dictionary (CancerWEB)]

Abrupt increases in fasting levels of plasma glucose concentrations between 5 and 9 a.m., in the absence of antecedent hypoglycaemia; occurs in diabetic patients receiving insulin therapy.

DCCT

The Diabetes Control and Complications Trial (DCCT) studied the effects of tight blood sugar control on complications in Type 1 diabetes. Patients treated for tight blood glucose control had an average HbA1c of approximately 7 percent, while patients treated less aggressively had an average HbA1c of about 9 percent. At the end of the study, the tight blood glucose group had dramatically less kidney disease, eye disease, and nervous system disease than the less aggressively treated patients.

diabetes (diabetes mellitus) - please refer to chapter "Diabetes Definition"

Diabetes is a life-long disease of high blood sugar caused by too little insulin, resistance to insulin, or both.

diabetic [Merriam-Webster's Collegiate® Dictionary]

n.: a person affected with diabetes

diabetic coma

A state of unawareness or loss of consciousness with a lack of ability to respond. Can be caused by either hypoglycemia or hyperglycemia.

exchange [JRB]

A serving of food that contains known and relatively constant amounts of carbohydrate, fat, and/or protein. The food used in an exchange is usually weighed or measured. The exchanges are divided into several groups: milk, fruit, meat, fat, bread, and vegetables.

For complete exchange lists refer to the American Diabetes Association website searching for Exchange Lists.

fasting blood glucose

FBS; Blood sugar levels; Fasting blood sugar

This test is used to evaluate glucose (blood sugar) levels. It may be used to diagnose diabetes, monitor diabetic control, or as a screening test.

Nothing By Mouth (NBM) eight hours prior to early morning testing.

fluorescein scan [Merriam-Webster's Collegiate® Dictionary]

Fluorscein is a yellow or red crystalline dye with a bright yellow-green fluorescence in alkaline solution - injected into a vein fluorescein is used to highlight and take photos of proliferated blood vessels in the retina.

gestational diabetes - see also chapter "Diabetes Definition"
...high blood glucose at any time during pregnancy

glucagon
Glucagon levels may be measured in persons with chronically or repeatedly low blood sugar (glucose) levels.

Glucagon is a peptide (protein) hormone that is released from the pancreas. The main function of glucagon is to stimulate the liver to release glucose between meals (glucose is normally stored in the liver as glycogen), and release of amino acid (alanine) from muscles. Glucagon also increases fatty acid release from adipose (fat) tissue and synthesis of glucose (from lactate or amino acids) in the liver. As the level of glucose is decreased, glucagon secretion from the pancreas increases, and vice versa.

glucolysis [Merriam-Webster's Collegiate® Dictionary]
the enzymatic breakdown of a carbohydrate (as glucose) by way of phosphate derivations

glucose
Glucose is a major source of energy for most cells of the body. Some cells (for example, brain and red blood cells), are almost totally dependent on blood glucose as a source of energy. The brain, in fact, requires that glucose concentrations in the blood remain within a certain range in order to function normally

glucose tolerance - see glucose-tolerance test

glucose-tolerance test

Glucose is the sugar that the body uses for energy. Patients with diabetes mellitus have high blood glucose levels. Glucose tolerance tests are one of the tools for making the diagnosis of diabetes.

The most common glucose tolerance test is the oral glucose tolerance test (OGTT). After an overnight fast, a patient drinks a solution containing a known amount of glucose. Blood and urine are obtained before the patient drinks the glucose solution, and blood is drawn again every hour after the glucose is consumed for up to three hours.

glycogen

Glycogen is glucose in storage form in the liver. It may be broken down to form blood glucose during an insulin reaction or during a fast.

glycohemoglobin - see Hb A1C

glycosolated hemoglobin - see Hb A1C

gram [JRB]

1 pound [16 ounces] equals 453 grams

Hb A1C

Hb A1c; Hemoglobin - glycosylated; GHb; Glycohemoglobin; Diabetic control index This test is used to measure blood sugar control in individuals with diabetes mellitus.

In normal individuals a small percentage of the hemoglobin (Hb) molecules in red blood cells become glycosylated (that is, chemically linked to glucose). Glycosylated hemoglobin can be separated from normal HbA by electrophoresis (a laboratory technique) into 3 fractions called HbA1a, HbA1b, and HbA1c. Normally only HbA1c is quantitated. The percent of glycosylation is proportional to time and to concentration of glucose. In other words, older red blood cells will have a greater percent of GHb and poorly-controlled diabetics (with periods of time where they have high concentrations of blood glucose) will have a greater percent of GHb.

health-care team [JRB]

The group of professionals who help manage diabetes and which may include a physician, registered dietitian, and certified diabetes educator, ophthalmologist, podiatrist endocrinologist or other specialists.

hyperglycemia [MEDLINEplus -MedicineNet.com Medical Dictionary (MedicineNet, Inc.)]

A high blood sugar. An elevated level specifically of the sugar glucose in the blood.

The term "hyperglycemia" comes from the Greek "hyper-" = high, over, beyond, above + "glykys" = sweet + "haima" = blood. High sweetness (sugar) in the blood.

hypoglycemia

Insulin shock; Insulin reaction; Low blood sugar

Hypoglycemia occurs when your body's blood sugar, or glucose, is abnormally low. The term insulin shock is used to describe severe hypoglycemia that results in unconsciousness.

IMHO [JRB] In My Humble Opinion

insulin

Insulin is a hormone released from the beta cells of the pancreas. Insulin's most important function is to facilitate glucose uptake by a variety of tissues, especially adipose (fat) and skeletal muscle. Insulin also stimulates the synthesis and storage of triglycerides and proteins.

Insulin is the most important regulator of blood glucose. High blood glucose (such as exists shortly after a meal) stimulates the release of insulin, whereas low blood glucose levels inhibit insulin release.

insulin-dependent diabetes mellitus (IDDM) - see Type-I Diabetes

insulin reaction - see hypoglycemia

islets of Langerhans - see pancreas

isophane insulin
NPH (neutral protamine Hagedorn) insulin, a neutral pH, intermediate-acting insulin.

Joslin, Elliott P (Proctor), 1869-1962 [Michael Bliss's The Discovery of Insulin]
Elliott Joslin ['the master clinician of diabetes' who worked at the time of insulin's appearance] devoted his life to the treatment of diabetes. He also realized that the disease was far from solved by insulin. He considered insulin the end of one era in diabetes management, not the end of diabetes.

"It has been forced upon me that diabetic gangrene is not heaven sent but earth born."
E.P. Joslin 1934 (61)

juvenile diabetes - see Type-I Diabetes
Now called Type-I or insulin-dependent diabetes mellitus (IDDM).

ketones

Ketones (beta-hydroxybutyric acid, acetoacetic acid, and acetone) are the end-product of rapid or excessive fatty acid breakdown. As with glucose, ketones "spill over" into the urine when the blood levels are above a certain threshold. Fatty acid release from adipose tissue is stimulated by a number of hormones including glucagon, epinephrine, and growth hormone. The levels of these hormones are increased in starvation, uncontrolled diabetes mellitus, and a number of other conditions.

metabolism

Physical and chemical processes within the body related to body functions. Processes of energy generation and use; including nutrition, digestion, absorption, elimination, respiration, circulation, and temperature regulation.

mg/dl (milligrams per deciliter) [JRB]

The unit of measure used to describe blood-glucose levels.

ophthalmology [Merriam-Webster's Collegiate® Dictionary]
(see also retinopathy)

a branch of medical science dealing with the structures, functions, and diseases of the eyes

optometry [Merriam-Webster's Collegiate® Dictionary]

the art or profession of examining the eye for defects and faults of refraction and prescribing correctional lenses or exercises

pancreas

An organ called the pancreas makes insulin. The role of insulin is to move glucose from the bloodstream into muscle, fat, and liver cells, where it can be used as fuel. People with diabetes have high blood glucose. This is because their pancreas (islets of Langerhans) does not make enough insulin, or their muscle, fat and liver do not respond to insulin normally, or both.

photocoagulation [Merriam-Webster's Collegiate® Dictionary]

a surgical process of coagulating tissue by means of a precisely oriented high-energy light source (as a laser)

regular insulin

Regular or short-acting insulin (human) usually reaches the bloodstream within 30 minutes after injection. It peaks anywhere from 2 to 3 hours after injection, and is effective for approximately 3 to 6 hours.

retina

Internal layer of the eye that receives and transmits focused images. The retina is normally red due to its rich blood supply. It can be seen with an ophthalmoscope, which allows the examiner to see through the pupil and lens to the retina. Changes in color of the retina or changes in the appearance of retinal blood vessels may indicate disease. Changes in color perception and in vision also indicate disease and indicate the need for a retinal examination.

retinopathy (see also photocoagulation)

Disease of the retina. Retinopathy occurs in persons with prolonged, poorly controlled diabetes and involves abnormal growth of and bleeding from the capillary blood vessels in the eye.

self-monitoring of blood glucose (SMBG)

A technique of testing a person's blood-glucose level in order to determine the body response to activity, food, and medication.

subcutaneous
Beneath or under the skin. Cutaneous means of or in the skin.

sugar - see also carbohydrates
Glucose is the sugar that the body uses for energy.

Type-I diabetes - see also chapter "Diabetes Definition"
[Insulin Dependent Diabetes Mellitus (IDDM)]
...usually diagnosed in childhood. The body makes little or no insulin, and daily injections of insulin are required to live. Without proper daily management, medical emergencies can arise.

Type-II diabetes - see also chapter "Diabetes Definition"
[Non-Insulin Dependent Diabetes Mellitus (NIDDM)]...
...far more common ([than Type-I Diabetes] - about 90% of all diabetes cases) and usually occurs in adulthood. The pancreas does not make enough insulin to keep blood glucose levels normal, often because the body does not respond well to the insulin. Many people with Type 2 diabetes do not even know they have it, although it is a serious condition. Type 2 diabetes is becoming more common due to the growing number of older Americans, increasing obesity, and a lack of exercise. Without proper management, long-term health risks such as heart disease, stroke, and kidney failure can occur.

John R. Bennett

Acknowledgements

First and foremost, I give praise to my Mom for her patience and her caring. To my wife and children for their support. To Heather and Joshua, my grandchildren, who consistently raise my ego.

Thanks to Marcia Swiss, a coworker at Brookhaven National Laboratory (BNL) for proofreading my manuscript, John Woodworth, MD and Rev. James Bennett for their editing and many invaluable suggestions.

Thanks to Dotty Stevens, my Diabetes Educator, Paul Kessler, a retired (I'm envious) coworker at BNL and Sue Sevian, a *current* coworker at BNL for their testimonials. All three are extra special personal friends, as well.

Thanks to the following companies who have given me permission to reprint numerous photos.

- ◆ Becton Dickinson, Company
- ◆ Eli Lilly
- ◆ Medtronic MiniMed - Medtronic Minimed, Sof-set, Sof-set Micro QR and Paradigm are registered trademarks of Medtronic MiniMed, Inc.
- ◆ LifeScan - LifeScan, Inc., a Johnson & Johnson company

I especially want to thank Paul Madden, Special Assistant to the President, Joslin Diabetes Center for his praise of this book and for the years of our friendship.

John R. Bennett

Diabetes Definition

Excerpts   from: MEDLINEplus www.nlm.nih.gov/medlineplus/dictionaries.html a web version of "U.S. National Library of Medicine (NLM), 8600 Rockville Pike, Bethesda, MD 20894".

*   *   *

Diabetes is a life-long disease of high blood sugar caused by too little insulin, resistance to insulin, or both.

To understand diabetes, first consider the normal process of food metabolism. Several things happen when food is digested:

A sugar called glucose enters the bloodstream. Glucose is a source of fuel for the body. An organ called the pancreas makes insulin. The role of insulin is to move glucose from the bloodstream into muscle, fat, and liver cells, where it can be used as fuel. People with diabetes have high blood glucose. This is because their pancreas does not make enough insulin, or their muscle, fat and liver do not respond to insulin normally, or both.

There are three major types of diabetes:

Type 1 diabetes, which is usually diagnosed in childhood. The body makes little or no insulin, and daily injections of insulin are required to live. Without proper daily management, medical emergencies can arise.

Type 2 diabetes, which is far more common (about 90% of all diabetes cases) and usually occurs in adulthood. The pancreas does not make enough insulin to keep blood glucose levels normal, often because the body does not respond well to the insulin. Many people with Type 2 diabetes do not even know they have it, although it is a serious condition. Type 2 diabetes is becoming more common due to the growing number of older Americans, increasing obesity, and a lack of exercise. Without proper management, long-term health risks such as heart disease, stroke, and kidney failure can occur.

Gestational diabetes, which is high blood glucose at any time during pregnancy.

Diabetes affects 16 million Americans. There are many risk factors for diabetes, including:

Family history of diabetes (parent or sibling)
Obesity
Age greater than 45 years
Certain ethnic groups (African-Americans, Hispanic-Americans)
Diabetes during pregnancy or baby weighing more than 9 pounds
High blood pressure
High blood levels of triglycerides (a type of fat molecule)
High blood cholesterol level
The American Diabetes Association recommends that all adults be screened for diabetes at least every three years. A person at high risk should be screened more often.

Maintaining an ideal body weight and an active lifestyle may prevent the onset of type 2 diabetes.

Currently there is no way to prevent type 1 diabetes.

High blood levels of glucose can cause several problems, including frequent urination, excessive thirst, hunger, fatigue, weight loss and blurry vision. However, some people with high blood sugar experience no symptoms at all. About 40% of Type 2 diabetics have no symptoms of their condition.

Symptoms of Type 1 diabetes:

Increased thirst
Increased urination
Weight loss in spite of increased appetite
Fatigue
Nausea
Vomiting

Symptoms of Type 2 diabetes:

Increased thirst
Increased urination
Increased appetite
Fatigue
Blurred vision
Slow-healing infections
Impotence in men

Patients with Type 1 diabetes usually develop symptoms over a short period of time, and the condition is often diagnosed in an emergency setting. In addition to having high glucose levels, acutely ill Type 1 diabetics have high levels of ketones. Ketones are produced by the breakdown of fat and muscle, and they are toxic at high levels. Ketones in the blood cause a condition called "acidosis" (low blood pH). Urine testing detects both glucose and ketones in the urine. Blood glucose levels are also high.

Type 2 diabetes is diagnosed when:

The blood glucose is 126 milligrams per deciliter (mg/dl) or higher on two occasions after fasting (abstaining from food) for 8 or more hours; or

The blood glucose level is 200 milligrams per deciliter or higher at any time between meals with symptoms of diabetes, such as increased thirst, urination, and fatigue; or A blood glucose level drawn two hours after drinking a 75-gram glucose solution is 200 milligrams per deciliter or higher.

The hemoglobin A1c (HbA1c) level is a measure of average blood glucose during the previous two to three months. It is used to monitor a patient's response to diabetes treatment.

Blood sugar testing, also called "self-monitoring," is done using a special meter called a glucometer to check the amount of glucose in a drop of blood. Testing is usually done before meals and at bedtime, though more frequent testing may be needed during times of illness or stress. If it is done on a regular basis, testing informs the diabetic patient and their healthcare provider how well diet, exercise, and medication are working together to control their diabetes.

Blood sugar testing results can be used to adjust meals, activity, or medications to keep blood sugar levels within an appropriate range. They allow healthcare providers to recommend changes in diabetes treatment. Testing will identify high blood sugar and low blood sugar levels before serious problems develop.

Ketone testing is a second test that is used in Type 1 diabetes. Ketones build up in the blood when there is not enough insulin in Type 1diabetes and eventually "spill over" into the urine. The ketone test is done on a urine sample. High levels of blood ketones may result in a serious condition called ketoacidosis.

About the Author

John Bennett is an active, healthy fifty-three year old who just happens to have insulin dependent diabetes. Since the age of six, he has successfully and enthusiastically met every challenge that either his diabetes or normal life challenges keep throwing at him. An avid bicyclist and kayaker, he thrives on physical exercise; as a computer analyst writing scripts and creating web pages, he enjoys earning his living; as a Christian he testifies to having a 'living faith'. John considers that nearing fifty years with insulin dependent diabetes makes him an expert on the subject. He is a proponent of the insulin pump combined with frequent blood sugar testing. He's always reading and studying new innovations designed to combat his disease. Along with his daughter, who also has insulin dependent diabetes, he believes that the cure for diabetes is still within his lifetime.